MW01107767

# I Wrote a Book About It...

Gerry Martin

Ajoyin Publishing
P.O. Box 342
Three Rivers, MI 49093
Ajoyin2014@gmail.com
1-269-273-3600

I Wrote a Book About It
ISBN 978-1-60920-140-1
Printed in the United States of America
© Gerry Martin
All Rights Reserved

Library of Congress Number in process

API
Ajoyin Publishing, Inc.
P.O. Box 342
Three Rivers, MI 49093
Ajoyin2014@gmail.com

I SPENT THE BETTER PART OF the last thirty-six years attempting to have short stories, poetry, children's stories, or nonsense literature published to no avail. So now that I am a retired man that spent thirty-six years working to protect public health, I will be again testing the waters endeavoring to have my written word published.

I have always enjoyed the world of puns and jokes. I might have been influenced by my uncle Will or by my cousin Norm. They both could tell a story or joke and make everyone laugh. As I recall, there was not a dark side to the stories or jokes. The stories, most of the time, were based on true occurrences. The jokes and stories could be told in mixed company and in front of children. However, those were the days of Jack Benny and Red Skelton, when four-letter words were not needed constantly to create humor.

I have been told many times that I should write a book on some of the stories I have related about my life and my job. So if you are reading this, I have accomplished my intentions a book for my children and grandchildren to keep in their archives.

Most of the time, I will not mention names of people or specific towns or cities, because the characters and locations could be found in anywhere in the midwestern United States. The names are left out to protect their privacy.

My first thirteen years of life were spent on a farm that spanned eighty acres. About sixty acres of land were used for production of crops. The remaining portion of the land contained a two-acre portion of lumber, a small orchard, two acres of wetland, buildings, grassland and a driveway. The farm bordered the northeast corner of two country roads. My father was not unlike most young farm boys of his times. He worked as a laborer for other farmers until he earned enough money to make a sizable down payment on his own farm and to marry my mother. He and my mother knew they would spend the next years raising a family and trying to get ahead.

I was not unlike any John Smith who lived in a rural area in those days in the state of Michigan. I could not be John Doe, because no one knows John Doe.

My poetry and nonsense will be scattered among my tales and book chapters. Therefore, I will begin with a poem about my favorite individual sport, golf. This poem is about my life, told as a fractured nursery rhyme. This will provide an initial idea of things to come within this book.

# The Object of My Affection

Chasing around the object with a bag of instruments, a task
sounding similar to that of a physician or a mechanic.
Sodbusting can occur occasionally or frequently.
Trapping also can enter the equation, since the size of the pelt of
turf can be rather substantial.
However, good sportsmanship requires that the pelt not be left to
die, but be returned to its original state as nearly as possible.
Using the foot to tamp the edges down can prove to be
advantageous, unless, of course, the foot has been temporarily
injured by kicking a solid object.

Trees and water, although great for beauty during different
seasons, can prove to be less functional for the participant.
Purposeful lawn care can cause an obstacle for attacking the
object.
This can be troublesome.
These impediments many times provide a source for a rousing
game of hide-and-seek the prize for finding the hidden object
being the ability to hit the object again.
Not finding the object is very harsh; you must be penalized with a
pass at the object without actually attempting a strike at it.

Finding a ball behind a tree or at the edge of the water can use
your croquet or polo skills.
An implement which can be found on your person can be used. .
. .
The foot or the hand wedge, however, are illegal to use and can be
a blow to your character if you are caught using either process.

Dodging flying objects can prove to be stimulating and keep you
aware of your surroundings.

It is customary to yell "fore" if you have caused the object to propel toward another competitor-"fore" meaning to watch out, duck, or hit the deck (not the number of individuals you have struck in a day).

In most cases the aftermath of the yelling will be followed by a yell of "Thanks," "O.K.," or a friendly wave.
However, sometimes your kissing-up skills are needed if this does not Work, to avoid needing to use your boxing or wrestling skills.

Your wading, tree-climbing, and fishing skills may be needed should you need to retrieve an object from water or tree locations.
Some individuals may need these skills after throwing an implement.
But this is in no way part of proper sportsmanship.

Usually the club thrower is not up to par to start with.
The individual becomes teed off at the drop of an opponent's putt.
He or she carries a chip on his or her shoulder until they become green in the face.
They do not play the fairway, and make it rough for others.

Being able to drive a vehicle is not mandatory but helps you get to the field of play more readily.
Sending the object in a straight line will make one an excellent driver who can drive or walk to the object without tribulation.

If you walk through the playing field, it is recommended you bring an extra pair of shoes and socks just in case you get a hole in one.
You may see several birdies in a day.
Eagles are rare, and an occasional goose may be seen.
If you are near water, you may see a seagull. It is hard to shoot a birdie, though, when on the beach.

The game is golf.
If you do not have too many irons in the fire, you can join a golf club.
Joining a club is the object.

# A Place Called Peace and Love

Look how the light from the morning sun says no more
Isn't love of life what we need to know?
Followed when we are young
Tens of thousands of people will leave this world,
But love of life is what we live to know
Love brings you home again.
Men play cards in the tavern in a farming town
It is winter there
When they lose they do not complain
They just play again
These are friends, neighbors, and relatives from way back
Boy cousins and friends
Tease girl cousins and friends
That, when they grow up, they dearly treasure and adore
They dance around a bonding fire that bonds them
Family reunions and town gatherings light up the summer days
and nights
Singing songs of delight

# Fairy Tale Fractured

Humpty Dumpty had a great fall.
He spent his winters trying to gather himself together again.
In the spring he played the shell game;
In the summer he fried.

Old King Cole was a merry old soul,
But the kingdom took its toll on him.
He became grumpy some,
Being less fun.
Of course he was always under the gun;
It got so bad people started calling Attila the Hun.
Hearing this in jest,
Wanting the best,
He contemplated on top of a knoll.
He became a poor soul.

Peter, Peter, pumpkin eater
Trims his patch with a weed eater.
He was not his brother's keeper,
Therefore he made some wine.
The wine was fine,
But his brother became pie-eyed.

Jack and Jill went up the hill.
They found a nice home,
No more to roam.
They still live there with their son Will.

Jack be nimble,
Jack be quick.
Jack went through poison oak,

The poor bloke.
Jack developed a rash on his legs.
Jack wasn't nimble or quick.
Jack got burnt by a candlestick.

May had a little lamb;
His name was Sam.
He went to school one day.
He got in a jam
For being a ham;
He went on the lam.
Mary, after many months, found Sam.
Sam was no longer a little lamb.

Merry Mary knew Con Terry;
Terry was in debtor's prison.
He stole a pig from Tom, Tom, the Indian.
Miss Muffet was supposed to be watching the pig,
But she was eating away at her curds.
Away ran Terry with the pig,
But the Farmer in the Dell caught him.
Bashful, the Dwarf Sheriff, arrested him.
And Hi-Ho, it was off to jail they went.
He spent his prison time with Old Hickory Dickory Dock,
Who was in prison for cleaning Ben London's clock.

Hiram Diddle was in a bluegrass band.
Folks just called him "Hi."
He lived in the mountains; he was a highlander.
Well, old Hi had a cat that lived in his fiddle.
One day a cow tried to jump over Hi's moonshine.
She broke his jug line.
Now Emma Witherspoon had a mighty fine line of shine,
So Hi went to buy some shine from her.
He took his three-legged, one-eyed dog named Lucky Sport.
Emma's own little dog laughed to see such a sport.
While Hiram was gone, Emma's brother went to visit Hiram's
sister.

She was a real looker.
They decided to elope.
So the dish ran away with a Witherspoon.

There was a young lady who lived in a rather large shoe.
The poor soul had so many children she did not know what to
do.
Her husband was a heel and would not work.
She was fit to be tied.
But she cheered herself up when she did laundry.
Finally she told him, "Work, or I will give you the boot!'
He found a job as a field goal kicker.
The family moved to a flat.
They made perfect music together.

Peter Piper had perfect penmanship.
Penny Piper collected particular pennies.
Paula Piper preached on a parapet and became parched.
Pedro Piper picked a peck of pickled peppers.
Perry Piper packed the picked peppers.
Paul Piper was plagued with persistent pimples.
He was persecuted, but he patiently persevered.
Patty Piper was a polite, passionate percussionist.
Pepper Piper played piano with perfect posture.
Philip Piper was a priest who prayed and preached the precepts
powerfully to a Polish precinct in Poland.
Pauline Piper wore purple peony loafers with a pink petticoat.
Porter Piper pinned up pictures of a pinto pony on a plaster pillar.
Patrick Piper prepared a paper to be printed promoting
purposeful purchases of property.
Polly Piper the parrot, so named, played upon her perch.
Preston Piper was a poised, polite, precise polo player.
Grandma Peggy Moses Piper painted pictures of porcupines,
porpoises, polar bears, and potent polecats.

Three optically challenged mice,
Three optically challenged mice,
Look how quickly they move for three handicapped rodents.

They smelled some cheese--
But where?
They all ran in different directions.
One ran after the Farmer's wife;
She cut off his tail with a jackknife.
The second ran into a hired hand.
He captured him and put him in a pumpkin shell,
And there he kept him very well.
The third ran into a man named Disney.
Mr. Disney had a vet perform laser surgery on him.
This corrected his blindness.
Then Elmer, as Mr. Disney was known, named Hi "George."
George was curious.
He traveled many years with Elmer.
One day while rabbit hunting,
George was with his tailless brother, Buggs Fudd.
George said, "Funny after all these years, you running into me."
Buggs said, "I been tailing you for some time."

Simple Sally Simkins
Met a pie guy
While walking through the rye.
Said Simple Sally to the pie guy,
"You have any cherry pie and some napkins?"
The pie guy said with a sigh,
"I have only apple and peach pie today."
Sally said, "I will take a bit of peach pie and make sure there are
no pits.
'Cause peach pie with pits is the pits."

Little Girl Red
Was sick in bed.
Little Boy Blue
Blew his horn.
Nurse Green
Said real mean,
"Blue, blow this town,
Or I will call Policeman Brown!"

Blue ran to the house of Bud Tan.
Bud was out back playing cards
In a field of corn
With a purple martin on his shoulder.

# The Sand Pit

MY FIRST FIVE YEARS WERE rather isolated. PlayStations and the internet were in the distant future. Good morals, common sense, and work ethics were the norm. My father and mother expected 100 percent effort in everything we did. Education was foremost for a better life than they had. Radio programs were our entertainment. Once or twice a week, homegrown popcorn and homemade grape juice were supplied for our evening pleasure. A few times we visited my uncle and aunt's home down the road to watch their Zenith television. In 1955 we were introduced to a Philco television set of our own. Most of the time we thought entertainment was playing in the woods; fishing; and pick-up baseball, football, and basketball games for older children. My first five years were spent playing with toys and once in awhile finding an outdoor activity. One of these projects went something like the following:

During the summer of 1952 when I was 4 years old, at some time or other my folks purchased a shovel and pail for me. Now the placement of our house was on the highest portion of the property. The barn might have run some competition with the elevation of the house, but I believe the house would win any discussion. We had an orchard of apple trees, pear trees, cherry trees, and a row of grapes. This orchard actually formed the border for our potato patch. There was a chicken coop and a shed used for the tractor and the garden. All of these areas were much lower than the house. A horseshoe driveway existed which formed a half-circle around the house. This went between the shed, chicken coop, and past the west end of the barn. A drastic slope existed at the east end of the house, which leveled off where the driveway crossed.

At the base of this slope west of the driveway, I decided to dig with my shovel and use my pail to remove soil to another location.

It started out rather innocently. When asked what I was doing, my parents were informed I was digging a gravel pit. My folks thought it was a cute idea. After all, it would keep me busy for a while, and how long could it hold my attention before I gave up? After all, a four-year-old boy could not remove too much soil.

This, however, became an everyday project. I continued for a week, removing soil to various locations. We had dry weather, so operations were not held up.

The second week, a dump truck I received from my godfather for Christmas was added to the process. Halfway through the second week, my uncle (who was a plumber and had the Zenith television) stopped by to visit. He commented on what a good job I was doing. Now this uncle was my favorite uncle at the time, to because he was always speaking of taking me to Big Rock Candy Mountain, where there was all the candy you could eat. So I was inspired even more. The operation then advanced to using a small spade and my red wagon.

On Tuesday of the third week, my dad, after my early arrival for work at the gravel pit, came from the barn after finishing his morning chores to halt the project. He had evidently surveyed the area more closely before he began the chores and had observed things had gotten out of hand. He tried to explain to me the reasons for placing the Stop Work Order on the project. I could not understand why it was a problem. A thunderstorm that night, which washed away more soil, brought the concerns more clear. The next day, my father replaced the soil; however, this continued to be a problem for some time when it rained. When I attended school, I learned more about erosion.

# Discipline

SITTING ON THE BOTTOM STEP of the stairway to the upper level of the house, with a closed door in front of you, became rather fashionable for punishment in my home. These tactics by my parents conventionally replaced the spanking of the times. This was Mother's futuristic thinking regarding "time-out" of today. Of course, my mother's conditions were more isolating. The duration of events appeared not to be consistent, although my mother must have had some sort of sentencing structure, but I don't recall unlocking the key to her methods.

The door and the stairs were your only friends for this period, and heaven forbid if you moved from the step, because an occasional checkup on your location was part of the process. I was once burned by this, by moving up and down the steps in a playful manner. Time in the "cell" was added. I will admit any time spent thinking over your offense was rather thought-provoking.

My mother and father had a special tone in their voice when punishment was in order. Any time I heard this tone and was stationed at the outer limits of our house, I headed for the cornfield when the corn was high enough to hide in or I hid where I could find the closet cover. The cornfield was the best when the season was right. I still received the stairway sentence, but it seemed to reduce the decibels of the voice when receiving the oral portion of the discussion regarding the wrong I had done. Sometimes reform school was mentioned when I was older. A threat of reform school seemed to be the last resort for parents of those days.

On one occasion, I was wrongly accused of breaking my sister's watch. I was placed in the cell. My sister was in school at the time of the accusation. When she came home, she admitted she accidentally broke the watch. Insult was added to injury when my mother told me that the detention was for the next time I got into trouble. The next time I went astray, I did not receive compensation, as I recall.

# TALE THREE

........................................................................................................................

# The Pretend World

URING MY FIVE YEARS OF isolation prior to attending school, I had very few playmates, as all but two of my cousins were much older, and I did not see those two very much. There were no kids my age in the neighborhood. I had a dog, Saint Bernard given to me by my godfather when I was three. The trouble was, I could not go near him because he always knocked me down. A nice doghouse came with him. He killed some of the neighbor's chickens, and Dad shot him.

As a result, pretend friends were needed. I had Oswald and Marie Hunker, who lived on Barnhill. Their house was a rock a short distance from the southwest corner of our barn. The top of the rock extended above the ground about two inches and was about twelve to fourteen inches in circumference.

I remember some discussion with my dad about the rock's removal, because little boys need to know such things. Erosion was again mentioned as a factor, but the rock was not hurting anything remaining at its location, hence the rock became the home for Oswald and Marie. You could say I had them living under a rock. This, of course, was before the term "crawling out from under a rock" was used commonly.

I would sit on the rock and speak a lot about news issues my mom and dad would discuss at mealtimes while listening to the radio. The radio was usually in the background most of the day. Some days I would discuss with the Hunkers some methods of treatment by parents regarding yours truly, which I did not think were fair. I remember specifically when Joseph Stalin died. My folks discussed thoroughly what the future might bring.

Detroit Lions and Cleveland Browns games were broadcast in my locale (mid-Michigan). (Carling Black Label broadcast the Browns' games, and became one of my beers of choice when I became an adult.) Sunday pro basketball and Saturday college games also caught my eye. Notre Dame football was of some interest; however, when they beat Oklahoma to snap their winning streak, then college football became a happening thing. Van Patrick broadcast the Tigers' and the Lions' games. Dizzy Dean and Buddy Batner broadcast the game of the week. Curt Gowdy broadcast pro basketball.

I watched the Tigers; however, they were not so good. During these times I learned to hate the Yankees, so the Brooklyn Dodgers and the Milwaukee Braves became my teams of choice. Their games were broadcast the most besides the Yankees.

The Lions and Bobby Layne were very competitive. There were no pro basketball teams in Detroit. The Fort Wayne Pistons did not move to Detroit until 1957. So early on, I was not exposed to them.

Probably this was the life of many boys who lived in rural areas during these time; they had their pro teams in their local and became interested in a team because of local broadcasting, newspapers, and magazines. Trading cards also exposed one to several players in all sports.

In my pretend world, I personally played on all the professional teams of my interest. I played baseball for the Dodgers before I was traded to the Milwaukee Braves. I do not remember why I traded myself, but I did love Hank Aaron. In the real world I was also partial to Al Kaline; however, my cousin, who was a year younger than I, took him as his hero on the Detroit Tigers, so I chose Charlie Maxwell.

Michigan winters, school attendance, and working with my dad cut short my time pretending football stardom process.

I played pro basketball in our barn with a cheap basketball and a makeshift hoop for the St. Louis Hawks against the likes of Bill Russell, Bob Cousy, and Bill Sharman. I played for the St. Louis Hawks because I really liked Willie Naulls, Bob Pettit, and Clyde Lovellette who played for them. They always seemed to have close games with the Celtics. We won the Championship in 1956 in my world; however, in the real world I believe they finished tied with the Minneapolis Lakers and the Fort Wayne Pistons, winning the Western Division in playoff, but were beaten by the Celtics for the NBA Championship.

The area west of our barn was my playground most of the time. The summer of 1956 (I believe sometime in the month of July), one of my baseball games was scheduled. It was a sunny afternoon, after attending church in the morning, eating dinner (our name for lunch in those days), and performing my chores. I set out to play a doubleheader. I was playing for the Dodgers, and we were playing the Braves.

The setting of the area was like most baseball arenas; however, the bases, pitcher's mound, and home plate were the only area without grass. I also set up a target on our large twelve-by-fifteen-foot sliding doors on our barn, which were behind home plate. If any imaginary pitcher (being me) or me as myself hit this target, it was a strike. I was the pitcher sometimes, and the batter sometimes, depending on the situation. Hitting the ball to the road was a home run.

The game began. Don Newcombe was pitching for us, and Warren Spahn was on the mound for the Braves. Newcombe (me, of course, simulating Mr. Newcombe) struck out the side. I was leadoff hitter. I hit a ball to center after throwing the ball in the air and hitting it. Rounding first base, I tripped over the cultivator attachment for our tractor, which had been stored there temporarily. My mouth hit a portion of this device, chipping my front tooth. I managed to stop the bleeding, but the game was over for me due to my injury.

A visit to the dentist did not provide any tooth repair, as my parents could not afford the expense of the repair. Dental insurance was not the norm in those days. Basically, I knew where this was going. In the past, to save money, teeth had been pulled and filled without any relaxing medication. The tooth remained a source of discussion by my peers for years until I was twenty-eight years old, and dental insurance was available at my means of employment.

The Dodgers did win the World Series that year in the real world. In my world, however, I assisted them.

In my imaginary world, I do not remember knowing about actions of prejudice or performing them. Hank Aaron, Don Newcombe, Roy Campanella, Bill Russell, and Willie Naulls were my heroes. It was not until we studied slavery and Jackie Robinson that I learned what being prejudiced meant. I remember when Roy Campanella became paralyzed from his accident; I was shocked and sad. After reading his book *It's Good to Be Alive,* he was even more of a hero to me.

# Girls' World

MY UNCLE FRANK WHO LIVED down the road, as I mentioned before, had three daughters close to my sister's age. My sister was six years older than I. We did not travel in the same circles most of the time. My sister and these three would get together often. Once in awhile they would decide to play kickball. This action took place at my baseball arena. Now most of the time when they came over, I would stay my distance, in most cases by mutual agreement. On some occasions, unkind words were exchanged, so staying clear was to my advantage. When kickball was on the agenda, though, I became an asset.

Five players were more efficient than four, and I became the designated pitcher. This asset only lasted for the duration of the game, which did not last long for four ladies who did not hold sports as a priority. Soon after, the unkind words became bountiful to drive the little fellow away.

The ladies also had some rules that did not match the playground rules I was accustomed using with boys in school. But because of my need to have someone to play a sporting event with, I accepted the rules and continued the farce with each session. One rule was I was not allowed to cheer for one team at any time during the event. Another rule was I could not catch the ball for an out as pitcher; only they could. There were other rules, but I tried to forget them, and have succeeded, I guess, in only remembering that it was a farce. I do remember my friends in school and I discussed the issue, and they expressed similar experiences regarding the play of the females of the day.

On another occasion, they were going to take a walk around the four-mile section. This was of interest to me. Therefore, I requested to also partake in this venture. This was met with strong opposition. My mother intervened, and the ladies were boldly told to allow me to accompany them. Once we began the journey, I was told to keep my distance. This, of course, was not in my makeup. I followed directions for a time, but many times I infringed on their space. After, I guess, one too many advances, we came to a bridge. The four ladies proceeded to lift me kicking and screaming partially over the bridge.

Years later, I realized it was only a scare tactic and that they had been careful not to hurt me in any manner, but at the time the threat was successful. I continued the trip at a safe distance. Just before we reached our destiny, I was told not to tell on them. This incident was never told to any parent. I learned to compromise many times under a variety of circumstances.

# Ḧonesty

A TRIP TO THE FEED MILL with my dad was always a fun time. In fact, a trip with my father anywhere was a treat, because I could ask all sorts of questions, and he would take the time to answer them as we were driving.

We visited two different feed mills in two different towns the same distance from our farm in two different directions. One was west of our house, and the other was east of our home. Available supplies, type of supplies, and cost of supplies dictated the need for visiting different mills. The mill in the town east of our home doubled as a train depot for dropping off large items ordered by catalog, such as furniture. Watching the train come in, bringing the new possession, was exciting. Imagining where it came from and how it was handled was most of the excitement. If you raised pickles, you could bring them to this feed mill to be graded and be reimbursed. This town was also where our family doctor had his office in his residence. An IGA grocery and a barbershop existed within this town.

Most of the time we went to the town west of our home, because this was where my mother did most of her shopping. This was where Dad did his banking. This town had a hardware store, another grocery, a car dealership, two service stations, a barbershop, and a post office. My uncle was the postmaster of this post office. A small dam provided energy for the mill.

In those days farmers could borrow money on their name to purchase seeds for planting, which would be provided in the spring and paid back after harvesting the crops. Going in the bank with Dad to borrow the money was also a treat.

Two of life's learning experiences and lessons happened in these towns. One day when I was about five years old, I went shopping at the grocery department store in West Town with my dad. We were going through the fruit and vegetable section when I grabbed a strawberry and popped it into my mouth. My father observed this and explained to me why I should not do that. He made me immediately go to the checkout and pay a penny for the fruit. I never again considered doing anything of the sort until about two years later.

At both the feed mills and some service stations, young boys and girls would receive a free candy bar or such at the time the bill was paid. This particular day at the East Town mill, Dad bought some feed, cracked corn, and some oyster shells for our chickens. He talked to some of the farmers for some time in the office area. The office was quite busy with people paying bills or buying other items within the office. My dad handed the money to the clerk, the clerk handed the receipt to him, and the next customer was waited on. No candy bar was provided.

What was I going to do? The candy bars were within reach. I had to work quickly but without being seen, I grabbed one. Dad and I left immediately. I pondered what I had done on the way home. Guilt was on one shoulder.

Rationalization was on the other shoulder. Guilt stemmed from the strawberry incident: my rationalization was that I had always been given a candy bar before this, and I probably would have received one had the clerk not been so busy.

After two days, I still had not eaten the candy. It remained in my dresser drawer, somewhat melted from the ride home. Finally, I admitted my transgression to my dad. My father had mixed emotions. On one hand he was proud that it bothered me, and on the other hand, he told me it still did not make it right. The next time we visited the mill, I had to explain to the clerk what I had done. The clerk told my dad that he probably did not see me, and I would have received the treat if he had seen me. My dad told him that might have been true, but I needed to learn a lesson. I continued to receive the treats routinely after that but never considered taking items under any circumstances.

# The Barber

I MENTIONED THAT THERE WAS A barbershop in both towns. My first haircut was performed at West Town. The barbershop had the flavor of most barbershops in the rural Midwest during the mid-1950s. A potbelly stove that burned wood existed near the northwest corner of the room. Men gathered around the stove during the winter months to tell stories and relate gossip while waiting for their turn in the chair. The barber's name was Bill.

Bill was a jovial man who liked to tell jokes and keep lively discussion going on a variety of subjects. My father commented that many times he thought Bill would take the opposite opinion to keep things exciting. Bill would always say to little boys, "Do you want all your hairs cut, or just one haircut?" Some boys did not know what he was talking about initially, but after he explained, the boys would say they wanted all their hairs trimmed.

Bill had a stroke in 1957. His personality changed. He became real caustic at times and used some nasty words when speaking. He was offended when my dad asked him to speak appropriately in front of young boys. Bill told him if he did not like it, to go to another barber.

After that, we went to the barber in East Town. He did not have the personality of Bill. He just cut hair and mumbled once in awhile, but Dad seemed to be able to get him to talk. They would talk about Christian principles.

Sometime in 1958 while we were shopping in the hardware store in West Town, Bill came into the store, went directly to Dad, and apologized to him. He told my dad that he had been out of line. He said that his apology did not mean he wanted only to have us come back to his shop, but it was important to him that my dad respected him again. Later in the day we heard from others that Bill had rushed out of the shop with a room full of customers. He saw my dad and me go into the hardware store.

He told the customers, "I have something I must do." After Dad heard this, he went back to the shop and told Bill he had always liked him and it had been hard to not visit his shop. On the way home, my dad told me you should always think highly of a person who asked another person for forgiveness. After that, we started going to both barbers. Bill was never his old self, but he was always cordial to my dad.

In 1960, Bill's health slowly deteriorated, and he was open off and on. My dad died in April 1961. We moved off our farm soon after to a larger town, where I visited a barbershop there. When I turned sixteen and received my license in 1963, I went back to Bill's shop. He was bent over and rather feeble. As he slowly cut my hair, he told me, "I always respected your dad. I thought the world of him." I told him what my dad had told me on the way home after that day in 1958. He just smiled. Bill died soon after that. For some time one of my thoughts for a profession was to become a barber. Bill influenced that.

# TALE SEVEN

## The Flower Bed

NOW OUR FARM WAS PRETTY much endowed with rich soil for planting crops. My dad, with the proper rotation of crops each year, maintained a very successful yield of corn, wheat, and oats for a variety of purposes. An excellent yield of hay for feeding our dairy cows was the norm each year.

The original builder of our house, however, picked a good location to construct. The location had very sandy soil, and the growth of vegetation was not the best. The area not far from the house produced an excellent lawn. Mowing the lawn, however, was the least accepted chore of the young man responsible for this labor. This may have been because mowing with a push-powered reel-type lawn-mowing device took great effort on the part of the human horse who provided the energy behind it. We also had a garden and our crops. However, the constant growth of grass was not welcomed by the chief groundskeeper.

The perimeter around the house was my mother's prime location for the placement of all her species of flower plants. She thought the flowers dressed up our home. Due to the barren soil, every year richer soil was transferred from another location to these beds. The source was an area that was saturated remains of chicken manure removed to fields in early April. (What are those black spots in chicken manure? Answer: more chicken manure.)

In spring of 1955, my sister and I were contracted to haul this topsoil to its new home. My dad, who informed us that only the top layer of six to eight inches was to be removed, plus no large holes were to be left, initially supervised the source site. Furthermore, if any deeper sections could not be avoided, they were to be smoothed off.

My wagon was used to transfer the soil. This wagon had been purchased for me for Christmas 1953. The summer of 1954, I decided to paint the brand new wagon gray, the result of a visit to my cousin's home where he had painted his brother's hand-me-down rusted wagon green. At the time, I was not informed of the rust problem. The planning stages began on the way home from my cousin's home and continued off and on until I fell asleep that night. An early morning rise, after my dad went to the barn to perform chores, was the first step. Gray was my only choice, because it was left over from a previous project inside our tool shed. The deed was done swiftly and, I must say, uniformly (I was always a better-than-average painter). The need for the swiftness was because I needed to be present to assist putting the cows out to pasture after milking had occurred. My mother discovered my masterpiece when she arose to prepare our breakfast. There was a great deal of discussion regarding why I chose to perform the deed. At this time, I was informed of the rust problem my cousin had had. The logic behind painting the brand new wagon remained a mystery. The logic, however, was discussed for several years at family reunions. Most times, it was pronounced a cute thing for a child to do.

This wagon was hence used for the many loads of soil to be distributed around our home. The location of the source was considerably lower in elevation than the house; therefore, toting the soil was a chore, pulling a loaded wagon uphill. Around 8:30 a.m., the workday began. A very short time for lunch was provided. About 2:00 p.m., my sister and I began grumbling regarding the amount of work we were performing. The complaining became more intense thereafter. My sister was afraid to approach the issue with my mother. Dirty looks toward our mother did not seem to concern her, although the slightest frown earlier had been cause for needed attitude adjustments on our part. The task at hand may have caused our nonverbal actions to go unnoticed. Finally around 4:00 p.m. after delivery of a load, I placed my hands on my hips and stated, "We have worked about hard enough!" My mother burst out in laughter. She said (much to my sister's surprise, who had cautioned me against making any comments), "Yes, I guess you guys can call it a day." This was again retold at family gatherings by my parents. My sister always remarked that only I could have gotten away with approaching the issue in such a fashion. However, my "cuteness" only went so far, and it was rare that she was ever in trouble with my parents or anyone else.

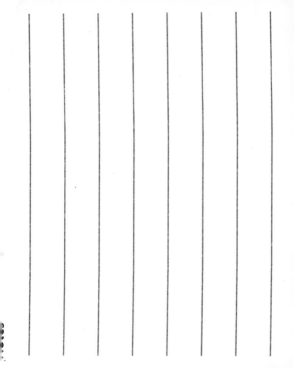

# TALE EIGHT

# Just Pa

MY FATHER WAS A MAN who was slow to anger. I only remember him losing his temper twice. The first was a mistake. The glass gas globe primer on our Allis Chalmers tractor came up missing one morning. I was in school attempting to complete my second year in school. A field needed plowing. I was nominated as the culprit to have misplaced it; I tended in early years to mess around with such items on occasion. Curiosity more than anything inspired me. Evidently my father was building up tension throughout the day, according to my mother. He stated something about waiting until I got home.

Dad met me at the bus which carried my sister and I to school and back each day. A rapid, continued slap on the butt guided me to the door of our house. He then explained his anger. In rebuttal, I explained that he had cleaned the filter the night before and placed the globe on a shelf in the shed where the tractor was stored. He agreed this had occurred, but said, "But it is not there now." We proceeded to the shed where, with some further exploration, we found the globe. It had fallen off the shelf to a difficult-to-spot location. Now, my dad was not a person to hug others. That day, however, a hug was given, with an explanation that jumping to conclusions was not in his makeup, but it had happened. Furthermore, the spanking was not normal for him, and he was sorry.

The next day, those who had witnessed my spanking gave me a rough time. Years later, it was still a subject to be discussed at social gatherings. Not wanting to make my dad look bad, I never discussed the misunderstanding in detail. Many knew of my dad's calm approach to life, and wondered what had happened to upset him so badly.

The other time my dad lost his temper was when he was trying to show my sister how to cultivate corn. She managed to remove several rows of corn in the process. I believe he was more frustrate than angry. For some reason, possibly because of my curious nature, I was nearby observing the disaster. The exchange between them was music to my ears. My sister never, ever did anything to get on the bad side of my dad (understandably, because she was basically well-mannered and respectful). I did, however, enjoy seeing her be in the hot seat for a change. This was very funny until the next day. My mother suggested that a young man halfway past his seventh birthday should become more involved with such farming procedures. Similar errors in carrying out these duties crossed my mind. Enjoyment of the incident the day before diminished. My fears, however, were replaced by my father's patience. I do not recall too much strife between us.

My father was a very pious man. He and my mother required us to recite the Rosary during the Advent and Lenten seasons of the Catholic Church year. He knelt down every night to pray before he slept. I recall he drove our tractor four miles and back to go to church and buy some food products when the roads were impassible for cars. One time he also drove the tractor to East Town and back to obtain medicine for my mother, who had had an asthma attack.

My father appeared to be a no-nonsense man. He did, though, have a dry sense of humor. One time my mother tried to get my dad's goat. We were sitting at the breakfast table, and she was pushing the issue that several successful men had found her attractive, and she felt many still did. After listening to this for some time, he said, "Well go, if you get the chance."

One day my dad and I were standing in front of the grocery/department store waiting for my mother to get done shopping. A man who only knew my dad casually approached him and demanded to know why Dad had burned down the shack he had lived in. This man, who had limited mental capacity, was a caretaker for a farmer who raised onions. (He once said a flat tire was not totally flat, only flat on the bottom. He was not trying to be funny.)

My dad proceeded to tell him he had no idea what he was talking about. The man continued to badger my dad until my mom had finished her shopping. After some investigation, my dad discovered that the man's shack had indeed burned while he was absent from the location. No one really knew how the fire started. Some young men, however, told the man that my dad started the fire. They picked my dad because he was the most unlikely person to do something of this nature. (Be aware that these were simple times; a prank like this was found to be fun.)

Once Dad found out what the situation was, he just let the prank ride itself out. A short time later the young men explained to the man what they had created. He did not really understand the purpose of the prank, and maybe rightly so. The burning of the shack remained a mystery.

Some of the young men who started the prank, along with others, assisted the man in erecting a new structure for him to live in. Once in awhile though, people asked Dad if he had burned any shacks down lately. He'd say, "Not recently."

We had a long row of Concord grapes that yielded more than enough grapes for our family. We ate them off the vine, and my mother made grape juice with them. Relatives on occasion would pick some grapes, as grapes were not available on most farms. Youth also stole grapes at times. If Dad heard them, he would yell, "Who is out there?" and they would scatter.

One Sunday after church, my dad decided to take a drive to observe some of the other farmers' corn. To a farmer, observing other farmers' crops in those days was equal to viewing the Grand Canyon, Niagara Falls, or the like. Taking a trip through the states of Kansas, Nebraska, or Ohio may have been boring to a person not in the farm profession, but to a farmer, this was a sight for sore eyes.

Two miles south, one mile west, and one mile south again of our home there was a burg I refer to as Southwest Town. This town had a tavern, two small grocery stores, a limited-mechanical-work service station, and a service station with major mechanical work available. A farm equipment supply store existed for farmers to purchase supplies readily. A pickle factory operated there for years before it closed in 1954. First and foremost, there was a Catholic Church, where 95 percent of the farmers attended Sunday worship; a parochial school where students attended until eighth grade; and a public elementary school which used a building owned by the church. All attended a high school operated through the school district. In 1962, a new high school and public elementary were completed.

Using a bicycle wheel for a description of the area surrounding the town--the town being the hub, and the spokes as the roads stretching outward five to six miles in all directions--these perimeters were the extension of the community. Beyond these boundaries, people were not as close. Most were German by nationality and chose the Catholic faith. The Eucharist ceremonies were attended each Sunday. Gathering outside the church during the warmer months after the ceremonies or gathering outside one or other grocery stores and sharing with each other was commonplace.

Approximately two miles north of our home was a store with a variety of items, but only one brand to choose from. They also sold ice cream cones. They had automobile fuel and oil available. An older lady and her son operated the store. They would check your oil for you. Occasionally you could receive a cone with an oil spot on it. This was, of course, frowned upon later in my life when I worked in the health field. In those days, I remember, for some reason it was accepted and at times joked about when you were lucky enough to not receive the extra flavoring.

On this particular day, we decided to stop at the store to purchase one of these cones. Now my dad most generally wore an old hat he had worn for years, bib overalls, a light shirt in the summer, and a flannel shirt during the colder months. This was the usual garb for a farmer. On Sunday, a farmer wore a suit and tie and, of course, a white shirt to church no matter what season of the year or what temperature. This respect for the visit to church is nowhere near this level today.

While we were waiting for our cones to be provided, three young men were commenting regarding an event they had participated in the night before. Stealing grapes from our farm was the subject. Laughter accompanied the belief that they had performed the deed without being caught. How they scouted out the area earlier in the day was also included in the conversation. Now, the store was located outside the borders considered to be part of the Southwest Town community. Apparently, the three boys had not ventured outside these borders very often. Therefore, my dad and the young men had not encountered each other very often. This, along with Dad being dressed in a suit, probably contributed to their discussion of the event at the particular moment. My dad approached the boys and informed them that he just happened to be the farmer who owned the grapes. Caught with their hands in the cookie jar, their emotions become apparent. After some words of apology, the boys shuffled out of the store, heads down and looking back occasionally prior to closing the door behind themselves.

My sister and mother had stayed in the car. When we joined them with the cones, Dad reviewed with them what had happened. He seemed to enjoy doing so. I do not think the three boys visited our property again. Fewer grapes were stolen after that as word got around about this encounter.

# Tale Nine

# Learning

RICKY NELSON WAS MY TEENAGE idol. I already spoke of a nice doghouse I received from my godfather. The establishment remained unoccupied for a number of years. My dad would mention once in awhile while we were doing chores that he might live there after a misunderstanding with my mother.

When I was both seven and eight years of age, two setting hens were placed in the unit to hatch fertilized eggs. It was my job to tend to the chicks after they were hatched. The purpose of this chore was to teach responsibility. Along the way I was also introduced to reproduction; at the time I did not have a clue. My dad told me at the time that a newborn calf "came down the lane," the lane being a fenced area leading back to our wooded area with gates to various fields. "Coming down the lane" both confused me and perked my curiosity. As most calves arrived in February or early March, I was curious to know how the calf, which I witnessed in a wet state, arrived on the premises and did not catch cold. Dad explained further that God took care of it until it arrived, then after its arrival it was our responsibility to take over the care. Later in life, of course, I learned the real story. I was enlightened as a result of playground discussions and actually assisting in birthing a calf. I always thought it was a big entitlement that God gave us to take care of this creature, until my children were born. Then I understood further what responsibility entailed for a living being.

Schoolboy discussions also provided the answer to why the bull we leased each summer acted in the manner he did, although some of the discussion needed updating and corrections as I got older, due to "misconceptions." This was explained to me as playing by my parents. Any discussion regarding the bull's use of his body part was greeted with, "You're too young to require any further explanation." Raising rabbits also contributed to my knowledge.

My father died when I was thirteen years of age. When I was about fifteen, my mother made an attempt at explaining the facts of life. I informed her that living on a farm and other sources had already exposed me to the subject. She seemed relieved that any further discussion would not be necessary.

One of the setting hens became so attached to her brood that they were almost fully grown, and she still had them gathered around her at night. When we finally placed her group with the rest of the flock, she wandered around alone and would not socialize with her peers. It was exciting watching the eggs hatch; the breaking out of the shell was amazing to me.

The doghouse had basically a flat roof with a ten-degree pitch. One summer, the flat roof became a stage. I had a number of sessions singing Ricky Nelson songs. I would use a badminton racket for a guitar. He recorded "Garden Party" years later. The stage was not too far from our garden, so you could say I had an early "garden party."

I thought the world of Ricky and his family. They were the American family. Mr. Nelson's life was an example of a boy placing a hero on too high a pedestal. I learned he was only human, and he had temptations like us all.

As I said, my father died when I was thirteen. The following is a tribute to him I wrote years ago.

# Ĥe Was Just Pa

He was born.
When his father's knee
Was a measurement for the corn
Everyone told his mother he looks like thee

Six siblings were happy he was alive
His year of birth was 1905
The family immediately glorified
The Supreme Being in the sky

His early life
Was full of strife
Emergency surgery almost killed him
His chance of survival for a short time slim

Prayer, faith, and love
Saved this young male dove
Other illnesses weakened his body parts
But did not weaken the love in his heart

He learned to love God
When by others he was shown
His guidance set the tone
For his faith and turning of the sod

He married his long-time friend in '41
The marriage was blessed midway
Before the setting sun
In the month of May

He had special relationship
With animals, seeds, and soil
Day and night, it was there he toiled
Fruit juices were all he would sup

A daughter was born in '42
In '47, another child
A boy came from heaven
At a time close to when Jesus was born anew

He never was known far and wide
But in love of God and neighbor he took pride
The moron and youth maybe made fun
Those who really knew him felt he was second to none

He died in '61
His daughter was a young woman
Early puberty for his son
His wife had trouble accepting God's plan

Those who had respects to pay
Had nothing but good things to say
A special man lived for his neighbor, his family, and God to pray
Left a big mark around a part of earth before he passed away.

# Tale Ten

# Pioneer Corn Cousin

ONE SPRING DAY, LIFE WHILE trying to complete my third
year of school was great. There was no evidence that trouble was
about to enter my world. I was laughing and joking with some of
my buds after a game of marbles. There was a willow tree in the middle of
the playground. I decided to pick a small sprig of a branch of this tree. As
I was talking, I was flipping this sprig. Out of nowhere my second cousin
appeared, and the sprig hit his ear. Evidently he thought I hit him with
intent. He began to cry. He said he was going to tell on me. I told him I
was sorry, that it was an accident. He ran into the school.

When he returned, he had the second grade teacher with him, Sister
Simon. Sister Simon was a tall woman who towered over most students.
You spoke only when Sister Simon said. I was told I was basically in trouble;
no explanation was requested.

Now my cousin and I did not travel in the same circles every day, but we
were related and maintained a friendship and played together occasionally.
There was never a misunderstanding between us prior to this. His dad was
my first cousin's husband on my father's side of the family. He sold Pioneer
seed corn. My mother's sister's husband sold DeKalb seed corn.

On occasion, at social gatherings, they were known to discuss what
seed was better. My cousin always said corn should be knee-high by the
Fourth of July. My uncle always said DeKalb corn was always butt-high by
the Fourth of July.

Sister Simon lectured about the pitfalls of hitting other children with
objects. I countered with "but, but, but . . ." That was as far as I got. She
said, "I do not want to hear your " 'buts' ." This, for some reason, caused
me to lose my temper in an uncharacteristic fashion. There were a variety
of Spritz balls for different purposes close to the area where Judge Simon
was holding court. I began to throw them on the flat roof of our school

until Sister Simon grabbed me and told me to stop. She pulled me along, taking several giant steps as we progressed into the school. My teacher, who belonged to the laity of the parish and seemed to have a little different manner of discipline, maybe as result of raising eight boys and one girl, was coming down the hall to meet us by this time. When we met, Sister Simon switched from holding me by the hand to pulling on my right ear while she explained her take on the incident. I had calmed down and remained mute. My teacher said she would take custody of me.

Silence from a teacher can be just as troublesome to a youth as verbal discipline. She said, "Have a seat, Mr. Martin, until recess is over." She left me alone for a bit and then returned without discussing the issue.

My classmates returned from recess, and no other communication occurred until the end of the day. At the time, it was customary that when you got in deep trouble, your parents and yourself would meet with the teacher before Sunday services to discuss the error you had committed. This was because farmers could not always drop their work to attend this sort of session on a weekday. A note was sent home with me requesting this visitation. The event occurred on Wednesday, so I suffered three-plus days contemplating what may happen, with tension at home at a premium.

On Thursday, my cousin and I discussed the issue, and he attempted to make amends with the teachers. He was stopped in his tracks with a comment that this was about me and not him. Therefore, no further discussion was allowed. As I remember, I was not treated any differently during this period.

Sunday finally came. We met in a room within the convent. In attendance were my parents, my teacher, Sister Simon, the principal of the school, and the accused--me. Sister Simon gave her views of the matter. After she finished, I began to speak. Sister Simon tried to interrupt me; however, much to my surprise, my teacher spoke up to say, "Let Mr. Martin continue." Our principal also agreed.

In those days, anger management consisted of your parents and teachers watching you like Elmer Fudd, "Very, very carefully." Your first offense was always with you during good and bad times, so second missteps were very rare. After that I had a real good relationship with my third grade teacher. I would say that she was one of my favorite teachers. Sister Simon and I never really became buds.

My cousin and I, as the years went by, would discuss this event along with two others that stood out in our memories. He and I had become closer as a result of "the balls on the school incident"; however, we still did not travel in the same circles every day.

The first episode happened when we were in eighth grade. It was the first basketball game of the season. When we were in seventh grade, anybody who came to practice could sit on the bench or play in a game. Sometimes there would be as many as twenty boys waiting in hopes of entering the game. Only seven or eight players actually played in the game. As the season went on, the attendance at practice dwindled. My cousin and I never gave up, but we still never played in an actual game.

When we reached eighth grade, standards changed. You could come to practice; however, only twelve boys were chosen to play or sit on the bench based on their effort in practice. This first game, my cousin and I were picked to be members of the group. I improved considerably to a point where our coach ranked me higher in status on the team. My cousin was a good baseball player and a better-than-average football player, but basketball was not his forte. He barely made the twelve. His hard work in practice was the only reason he passed muster.

The first game was an away game. We were getting our butts handed to us in the first half. Our coach, at halftime, proceeded to chew us out in the locker room. The yelling was rather intense. Finally our star player said under his breath, "Cool down, Coach!" This comment was not accepted well. My cousin was daydreaming with not a concern in the world because he figured he was the last person in the world to be considered part of the problem on the court. He was in close proximity to our coach, but out of line of his level of eyesight. Our coach turned to my cousin and said, "You go in the second half for Mr. Mouth there." Basically, the first person he made contact with was going in.

Anger had confused our coach's thought patterns. A sick look came over my cousin's face. You could see the fear in his eyes. Coach told us that he was leaving the room, and he wanted us to think about what he had said. While he was gone, my cousin went in the bathroom stall and threw up. Coach returned to lead us back onto the floor.

The second half started. Nerves and unfamiliar surroundings affected my cousin's quality of play. The ball was passed to him, and he threw the ball toward the basket as quickly as he received the pass. The ball somehow successfully went through the hoop. After that, it became ugly. His lack of defensive participation and general confusion on both ends of the floor led to his demise. He was removed from the game after two minutes had elapsed. The star replaced him.

We came back and won the game by one point. We always said if not for my cousin's basket, we would have lost. My cousin saw limited action after that, usually late in games when we were way ahead or way behind. That basket was the only points he ever scored. He went on to be a fair football player and a better-than-average baseball player in high school. He never participated in basketball during his entire high school career.

The second episode involved Sister Simon again. As I said, we were not buds. She kept a watchful eye on my actions as I progressed through school. A stern look was very effective when I made eye contact with her. However, she was the first nun to discuss my father's death after I returned the next day after the funeral when I was in seventh grade.

I had been appointed safety patrol boy the first day of school starting my eighth year in school. The job consisted of making sure smaller children were guided to the right bus at the end of the school day and helping the bus driver with any disciplinary problems. Each bus had one of these scouts, who were eighth graders. My cousin was also a scout. If disciplinary problems occurred, you reported them and a hearing was conducted every Friday afternoon.

One of the most difficult parts of the job, which I still remember as a tough decision in my life, was reporting my best friend, who challenged me to do so after he would not honor a request by the bus driver and myself to stop messing around and sit down.

The episode occurred just after I had been voted to play Saint Nick for the younger kids for treats on December 6. Next to being appointed safety patrol boy, this was the highest honor one could receive in the eighth grade. For whatever reason, which still escapes me, I decided just before the buses were to leave to run and extend my middle finger in jest to my cousin. This was a movement which occurred among boys periodically. I do not believe most boys really, at the time, knew the exact meaning of the gesture.

The next morning, I was greeted at the entrance of the school by Sister Simon asking why I had made the gesture. Furthermore, she asked me to explain the meaning of the action. I told her I was just fooling around, and after hesitating, I finally told her I thought it means, "Stick it up your butt." A jury of nuns proceeded to strip me of my job as Saint Nick. I still remained safety patrol boy, because my efforts on the job were commended by all.

I received a reprieve after my return from Christmas vacation. After considerable discussion, I was given a second chance. I was asked to be the back end of a camel for Three Kings' Day to pass out candy to children. Although the prestige was not even close to the Saint Nick job, it did get me out of class for a period of time. I got to place my face near the butt of the gentleman picked to be the front end of the camel. Imagine the pride I had in being selected for this job. Needless to say, I did not rush home to tell my parents of the honor bestowed on me. My cousin always told me he went to bat for me to get me the rear-end job, but he always snickered when he said it.

Vietnam called him; he served eighteen months there. He returned to the states and attended the same college that I did. He was killed in an accident the night before he was to be married. The last time we spoke, we discussed the basketball game incident and how scared he had been.

# TALE ELEVEN

## 𝕸oney 𝕸arketing

ID I MENTION I RAISED rabbits?
A shirttail cousin on my mother's side of the family became my first playmate on my first day of school. Both of us, for whatever reason, never attended kindergarten. It was never fully explained to either of us. All the other students knew each other from the past year. For three weeks we played together. Then one day I introduced him to a shy kid who rode on my bus. After a short period of time, two was company and three became a crowd. I became the odd man out. Our bonding ended abruptly when sand was thrown at me while completing my descent down a slide. My folks did not raise a dummy. I found companionship elsewhere with boys and girls who appreciated my company. These gentlemen maintained a lifelong friendship. A few months later, I returned to their company once in a while.

One day when I was in fourth grade, my dad dropped me off to play with my cousin while his dad and my dad went to an auction. During my visit, his brother introduced me to his rabbits. I further observed a miniature train village. His brother claimed he financed this village from raising the rabbits. This piqued my interest. I said, "You know, I bet I could make money, too, raising these animals."

When my dad came to pick me up, I discussed the issue with excitement in my voice. Responsibility to find the upfront money for developing the project was for me a pitfall for entering the business. Somehow, I convinced my dad to go along with my newfound plan for a source of money. We purchased two does and two bucks from my cousin's brother. The ease of raising these creatures, as described by the brother, became less apparent as the days turned into weeks. Cannibalism by the mother, immediately after birthing the offspring, and maintenance (feeding the rabbits and cleaning away manure) became a burden. I neglected my duties too much,

47

prompting my dad to threaten to remove them permanently from the premises. Dad wondered why he ever agreed to let raise rabbits because he ended up caring for them.

A number of times we sold the meat from the rabbits to a meat market. But the cost of raising them provided a very small profit. We would cut off their heads, skin them, and take them immediately to the market. Then one day the owner of the market said we needed to provide the carcass with the head left on (new requirement by the inspection agency who licensed the market to buy only rabbits with the head attached). This was instituted because recently a business owner had held a promotional barbeque serving rabbit as the main course. The people raved about the taste of the entrée. However, later cats' heads were found behind a building where rabbits were purchased. This explained why the man who held the function obtained the large amount of meat for such a good price. He even commented to his friends about what a good deal he had received. I guess this triggered a guest to check further into the reason for the savings.

My dad felt that this was the last straw as per an already complicated process of delivering the meat. The remaining rabbits were butchered, and that was the end of my eighteen-month rabbit business. My shirttail cousin's brother convinced other kids to also get in the business. Looking back, I realized this was where he made his money. I could never sucker anyone into purchasing my rabbits for this purpose; my salesmanship skills were lacking. I never did get my train village.

I was always trying to find a manner to earn some money. I raised pickles the summer I was ten years old. My dad worked the soil in an area east of our orchard. This area covered about three-fourths of an acre of land. Together Dad and I planted the seed to grow the pickles. I hoed and pulled weeds when needed. I picked the pickles twice a week and placed them in burlap bags.

Every week we delivered them to the mill in East Town to be graded. Unfortunately, all the competition from the larger growers forced the grading to be very particular. The grading was very size-and texture-specific. The pickles were to be sent to a processor who also needed to set certain standards of product quality. Most of the time, four bags of pickles were culled down to what amounted to one and a half bags of accepted pickles. The accepted units provided a small profit. This was hard to understand at my age, because product quality was not my main concern; profit was.

My mom made a variety of types of pickles that year from canned to crock varieties. We also ate a lot of cucumbers that year. Roadside stands did not exist, because everyone in the area raised their own pickles in their garden. My profit margin did not get me in a pickle again.

Collecting long-necked beer bottles tossed out of vehicles provided my best earning, because there was not any investment, only the effort of foot labor canvassing the roads. This was good until the return fee was lifted.

Taverns in those days were the only establishments that sold takeout beer. The tavern would give you a container which had small compartments for each bottle. You filled the container after the bottles were washed, and once filled brought it to the tavern to receive two cents per bottle for your efforts. This did not excite my dad, because he did not drink alcoholic beverages. Most people knew this; therefore, if anyone saw us go in or come out of the tavern, they would tease my dad, questioning whether he had taken up drinking.

My territory consisted of one-half mile east, one-half mile west, one-half mile north, and one-half mile south of our home. Once I expanded my area to an area one mile west and one mile north of our home. A fellow who frequented taverns told my dad I was infringing on his territory, and I better stay out of it. I honored his territorial rights, although Dad and Mom commented that he should stop drinking if he did not have the money to buy alcohol.

# TALE TWELVE

# Horse Tails

MY GRANDFATHER WAS BORN IN 1862; my father was born July 5, 1905; and I was born on December 12, 1947. This made for some interesting discussions when my children completed family trees for classes in school during the 1970s and 1980s. One teacher even requested proof of the birthdays of my grandfather and dad. My grandfather's first wife died in March 1899. There were five children born from this first marriage. The oldest offspring was born in 1886. His first wife, as she was dying, asked her friend to marry her husband when she died. Her friend did marry my grandfather. They married in November 1899. The second wife was my grandmother. This second marriage produced my dad, his two brothers, and one sister.

Horses were used to provide the "horsepower" to farm the land, before and many years after my dad was born. With this history, my dad therefore had an ingrained attachment to horses.

Until May of 1952, I had watched my father work behind a plow, hauling loose hay in a wagon to the barn, and using other implements with the horses. We had two horses for a long time. Their names were Barney and Doll. Then in 1950, Dad purchased a third horse named Dan for extra work when three horses were needed. This also rested the other two at times. I really liked Barney and Dan. Dan had a look in his eyes and his actions made you really like him. Doll was always aloof and skittish.

Sometime in March 1951, Dad came in the house and said Dan had balked out in the field. I had no idea what balking meant, but it sounded serious. Dad said once a horse balked, he was not worth a "plug nickel." I said, "What is balking, Dad?" He said it was when a horse will not move and should be working. He said, "Once a horse balks, you cannot count on it to work, and sometimes when a younger horse like Doll witnesses this, she may balk also." Dad said no two ways about it, we would need to get rid of Dan. I never really knew where Dan went.

One day in May 1951, I looked out the window and saw this truck coming down the road with a large object on the back. The truck pulled into our driveway and started to unload this object. I asked my mother what this large device with strange-looking wheels was. She said it was a tractor. I went outside to greet this new contraption. It had some letters on it which I learned to read: Allis Chalmers. I was told this was going to mostly replace Barney and Doll. Since Dan had decided he did not want to work, we needed more strength to use the implements we had. At three and a half years old, inanimate objects took on some sense of being similar to a toy. I did not like this thing with the name "Allis."

My dad told me years later that he too had liked Dan. Getting rid of Dan was one of the hardest things he had ever had to do, but a combination of Dan balking and the need to have the tractor to do work more easily caused him to take the necessary steps. He kept Barney and Doll "for small projects" he said, but I do not think he could part with the coworkers he had worked with for ten years.

Dad used Barney and Doll to gather logs for our wood-burning stove and to gather the remnants of hay and straw that were left behind by the hay and straw loader. He also used them to gather cornstalk bundles prepared by cutting down corn manually.

On one occasion when I was eight years old, we were gathering the remnants of straw on the edges of the wheat field. I was guiding the horses, who were pulling a wagon. Dad was throwing the straw onto the wagon with a pitchfork. A fly bit Doll, and as I said, she was skittish. She and Barney took off heading for a ten-foot-deep ditch which bordered the southeast portion of our farm. They stopped just short of the edge of the back of the ditch. The ground covered was two football fields. My father came running, which was a labor of love since he suffered from shortness of breath at times from a childhood illness. Gasping for breath he approached me a wide-eyed and scared boy. After some jubilation that the horses had stopped, we continued to work in the field.

That night while eating supper, we discussed the issue with my mother. She said, "Maybe if we still had Dan, he would not have moved." Since we were joking about the situation, I related that I noticed I believed both horses had pooped. I said maybe the horses were pooped out after their run.

One blustery and wintery day in early December 1954, a man was driving by our house. Suddenly he slid off the road. My dad collected Barney and Doll and brought them out to the area where the man was buried in the snow. Barney and Doll pulled him out. The man lived ten miles north of our home and raised Christmas trees. He told my dad that for his act of kindness, he could pick out a tree each year free of charge. We did this until Pa died.

Several years later in the 1970s a man ran off the road by my uncle's home. My uncle pulled him out with his tractor. A few weeks later, he received a letter from the man's lawyer claiming that my uncle had damaged the undercarriage of his car. The case never went to court, and the man never collected any compensation. However, it was an example of how times change and how gratitude can differ.

Barney and Doll were sold after Dad died to two brothers who lived down the road from us who also loved horses.

Although I never owned a horse myself, I still love the hayburners.

In my job as a health official, we followed up on nuisance complaints, which could cover a variety of health concerns. One day we received a complaint that someone had a horse in their barn that had died. I visited the residence in question. Indeed, a dead horse was found in one of the stalls in their barn. I told them they either needed to bury the horse with at least three feet of cover, or call a rendering company to pick the horse up. I told them the company probably would charge a small fee for disposing of the body. I also told them if they chose to bury it, they needed to place the horse in an area where higher ground existed and where the groundwater did not rise during heavy rains. They had a higher area a short distance from the house. I told them I would return in forty-eight hours to confirm what method they had used to dispose of the body.

I returned as promised, two days later. They directed me back in the barn, where I observed that the carcass had been buried in the stall where it had died with each leg extended approximately twelve to fourteen inches above the grade. The hoofs and the first joint of each leg were available for viewing.

My original intention was to steer the members of the family, which consisted of three boys in their late teens and their mother and father, toward having the rendering company pick up the animal. Digging in the area of the barn had to be a great chore, since the horses created a cement effect from daily movement atop the ground. The high area I had suggested west of the outbuilding would have been a much easier area to excavate with the shovels they had used to partially bury the horse in the barn.

After I witnessed this scene, I commented to them that this action in no manner matched my suggested methods of compliance for disposal of the horse. I told the family that I would again return in forty-eight hours to observe the proper removal of the dead animal from the barn.

I returned two days later, and they again directed me to the barn. The wizards had taken a chain saw, cut off each leg of the horse at ground level, and buried the portion of the legs in the same location, creating four small mounds of soil. At this point I shouted, "No, no, no! What are you thinking? This solution is more of the same." I returned the next day. They had finally took my advice regarding calling the rendering company. They dug the horse up, and the company took it away.

# The Postmaster's Wife

SOMEONE SAID ONCE THAT WHEN he asked his father what to do when the going gets tough, his father said, "Ask your mother. Don't ask me!"

My mother and my aunts were such women in the 1940s and 1050s. My mother, during those years, baked pastries every other day and cooked three meals a day. She washed Monday and Thursday each week with a wringer washer. A wringer washer had an agitator and a series of small rollers to wring the wet wash out when placed through them. The wash was hung outside on washlines during all seasons. In the winter, the wash was hung out to give it a fresh smell. Then the frozen wash was brought in and placed on racks behind our woodburning stove to dry. Mother cleaned the house from top to bottom each week using water warmed on our bottle-gas-supplied stove. This manner of heating water was used for washing dishes, taking baths, and washing clothes, as we did not have a water heater.

Mother washed windows inside and outside every month to six weeks during warm seasons. She canned vegetables throughout the summer and autumn from our garden which the family planted, hoed, and picked. She also canned fruits from our orchard: apples, cherries, pears, and grapes. She gathered eggs each day from our chicken coop. She made different varieties of crock and canned pickles. She sewed clothing from time to time. She mended socks and other clothing. She made quilts with the neighborhood women. Her flower garden was important to her to maintain.

Somewhere in between all of this, the washing needed to be ironed. The ironing was not a small task with the lace on dresses and other intricate layers on clothes. Bedding and underwear were also ironed. Helping my dad raise my sister and I was also in the cards. Raising me was a special chore in itself. My aunts and other women performed the same or similar chores and raised larger families.

I was amazed that mother had the time for pleasure, but she seemed to find it. Watching television only happened occasionally for Pa and Mother. My sister and I watched a bit more, but not an overabundance.

In those days, you had to get off your butt to change the channel. There were no remotes. One day my sister and I were watching television. It was rare that we ever did anything together. She told me to change the channel. I said, "Why don't you do it yourself?" to which she replied, "I told you to do so; you are closer." I proceeded to obtain a yardstick to measure who was closer. Indeed, she was found incorrect in her estimate.

My mother, seeing us being lazy, had a dictum, "You kids today are so lazy, you will be in wheelchairs by the time you are forty from lack of exercise." I did not realize my mother had been witnessing our discussion and my process in measuring. The statement regarding our laziness was included in her evaluation, including questioning why I could get off my dead butt to prove my sister wrong, but not to change the channel. I refuted that it must be because of my German heritage regarding being stubborn. That rebuttal seemed to satisfy my dad when she related it to him.

However, this statement did not set well with my mother. She countered with another of her locally famous statements, "You can have all the fun you want, but don't get funny." When this phrase was said, it inferred, "You better shut your pit hole, real quick." That ended any further discussion, and no confab regarding changing the channel for another person occurred in the future.

My dad's interest in sports did not go beyond tossing horseshoes. My interest peaked generally in sports when my aunt gave me some back issues of some sports magazines. I read these carefully.

Dad mentioned one time that he knew Charlie Gehringer, the Hall of Fame second baseman for the Detroit Tigers, when he was growing up. He met him when visiting his cousins who lived in his hometown. He also talked about schoolboy Rowe, who also played for the Tigers. When I showed little interest, he did not speak any further in their regard. Later, I learned of their stardom, but, unfortunately, it was after Dad had died. That, I believe, was the only time we discussed a sport of any kind. If I did comment about any sports subject, it was met with an "Oh?" and that was the only response.

The only source of fish we had was either from purchasing them at a store or when a neighbor dropped off smelt at our house during the spring season. Fishing was just not a part of our life. My aunt, however, who was my mother's sister and the wife of the postmaster from West Town, went fishing herself and taught a number of my cousins to fish. A month or so after Pa died, she took me fishing to a river a short distance from her house. My first experience was a great one. I learned what a mess of fish meant: twenty-one fish. This consisted of some bluegills and sunfish.

Digging for nightcrawlers for bait was fun. The excitement soon wore off a bit when I was told I had to clean my catch. My aunt showed me proper techniques on the first two fish from the mess. Then my shift began. Despite my fumbling around to clean the fish, my aunt did not volunteer to assist me. She only occasionally commented on where I was going wrong.

When I said that I had finished the task, my aunt's opinion did not correlate. She pointed out my deficiencies, and I returned to my duties at hand. After two more sessions, I met the acceptable standards. I took some of the fish home, but my aunt fried some of them. As I remember, they had to be the best fish I ever ate.

I returned many times after that and had rather good luck. I was also introduced to the species of fish my aunt called a bullhead. She always gave praise for my fishing skills and my ability to clean fish. The trial-and-error method of showing the proper method of catching and cleaning the fish was to my aunt's credit. She was a no-nonsense woman but was one of the kindest persons you ever wanted to meet.

My cousins (her three sons) said she could be impatient with them sometimes, but I never saw that side of her, nor did her other nieces and nephews.

My mother's father and mother were born in Germany. They met and were married in a small community in Michigan several miles east of our home. My mother, aunts, and uncles left a farm there in 1914 and moved to the area where my dad and mom grew up. German was spoken in the home most of the time. My postmaster uncle's parents were British, so German was not spoken much in his home, and my uncle and aunt did not speak German much either. It was a treat for my aunt when she visited with her siblings. Speaking German also came in handy when you did not want your children to hear or understand what you were talking about.

My mother babysat for different children overnight after my dad died. In one couple she worked for, the mother was originally from the

Philippines. Her sister visited occasionally, and they would speak in their native tongue. This would upset my mom, because she thought sometimes they were talking about her. I told her that she and my aunt talked in German in front of people sometimes who did not understand them. That was different, she said. They did not gossip about others. However, their idea of gossip was wide open to interpretation.

My aunt was a big Detroit Tigers fan. She did not watch much television. My uncle would watch the Tigers when they were broadcast, which was mostly on Saturdays. My aunt would listen to all the games on the radio. She listened until she died in the early 1980s. She loved every ball player and would never say anything bad about them. She did not like feisty Billy Martin when he managed the Tigers. She would say, "That Billy Martin, he is too wild-acting. Someone needs to talk to him like a Dutch uncle to calm him down."

You should not gossip; however, discussion sometimes can be boring if you do not speak of the latest news. There is a difference between "telling dirt on a person" or repeating hearsay or telling rumors that may only be half-truths and informing others of the latest happenings. I learned at a young age, five years to be exact, you must be sure of your source and must understand fully what you heard. My aunt and mother were talking one day about my uncle the postmaster's brother. I came into the room in the middle of their conversation. They said the brother married his sister. Being a little kid with limited thought patterns I mulled this over for a few days. Then I asked my dad what the deal was. He said, "Oh, Son, you know our parish priest is your uncle's brother. When his sister married her husband, he presided over the wedding." After some further discussion regarding the use of the word married, I understood.

My uncle could not see well later in life, and my aunt could not hear well. They traveled a lot all over the United States in an automobile. My aunt never learned to drive, so my uncle did all the driving. She was his eyes. She would ride in a car with her head about six inches from the windshield. Many railroad crossing in those days did not have audio signals, so they would stop at a railroad crossing and open the windows. She would look for the train, and he would listen for it. Riding with them was a trip in itself, watching them because your safety was always questionable. I don't, however, remember them ever having an accident, and they traveled thousands of miles, including driving to Florida and back each year.

My aunt never wanted to fly in an airplane; hence, they always drove everywhere. The year after my uncle died, my cousins convinced her to fly to Florida. After that initial experience, she flew everywhere. She turned into a frequent flier. Her oldest son said he knew she would enjoy flying once she did it, because she flew off the handle several times. My aunt did not appreciate that comment.

This son enjoyed the taste of amber fluid. He once told me that he did not have a beer before sundown, but the sun seemed to go down earlier each year, no matter the time of year. Another time he was visiting my aunt's farm. Where he lived in Wisconsin, it was about 10:30 a.m. He offered me a beer. I said it was too early. He said, "Nonsense; beer is like Wheaties, 'breakfast of Champions.'"

My uncle who fought in World War I lost a considerable portion of his hearing as a result of improper protection during the combat. After the war, he returned home and soon worked throughout the United States at a variety of jobs as a laborer. When he was older, he went to live in a soldier's home facility. He worked there for room and board at various projects. He would come home for a visit with his brothers and sisters once or twice a year. He also went on trips with one of his siblings once in awhile. He wore a hearing aid which had batteries that needed to be regenerated occasionally.

My uncle was a wonderful man, well respected by all his nieces and nephews. He told us stories of his travels when he visited each household of his siblings for one or two days. During his visits he would "rest" his hearing aids two or three times per day for reviving his batteries and the unit.

For a few years, facts that were private within a family seemed to become common knowledge to everyone in different families. My uncle was providing this information that all parties thought was being shared unrestricted. Each family could not remember sharing the data with him. Over time through a series of deductions, it was agreed that my uncle's hearing aid was not always "resting." Everyone began to watch what they said during the resting periods.

No one ever accused him of eavesdropping. He was such a sweet man and so enjoyable to talk to that it was not worth embarrassing him by approaching the issue. In addition, he seemed to enjoy sharing information since it made him feel part of everyone's family having been an unmarried man all his life. Sometimes I think at times he had a lonely life, moving from place to place early in life, and then living in a dormitory environment later. He never let on he felt forlorn, though.

Teasing can affect people differently. What is considered just kidding, joshing, or ripping to one person may be deemed harassment, taunting, ridiculing, and annoying to another. To one person, teasing may be just seen as innocent bantering; to others it may be overwhelming. How a person reacts to teasing depends on one's makeup or personality. Bullying can reach an overwhelming state for many children.

One day before I entered school, my sister came home crying. Some kids had sung a verse to her that went like this, "Mrs. Hart made some tarts on a rainy day. Mrs. Martin came a farting and blew them all away. This did not sit well with my sister and mother. Their grief turned to my needed discipline. I was not concerned too often with others' teasing. I rolled with the punches, so to speak. I learned early that if you appeared to be upset with teasing, kids would try harder to upset you.

My mom had nine siblings: six brothers and three sisters. My aunt was a twin. One day when both were close to two years of age, my grandma was picking pickles in a field. Some of the older children were assisting my grandmother. The others were playing randomly (my mother was not yet born at the time). It was hot and humid. My aunt's twin was nibbling slowly on a pickle. Evidently a short time later after she started chewing on the pickle, she began having trouble breathing. My grandparents rushed her to the doctor, but it was too late and she died.

The doctor and family never really knew what caused her death. She had been perfectly healthy before the tragedy. They blamed it on poisoning from the pickle. After that, the whole family never ate raw pickles in any manner. Even their children and grandchildren were not given pickles prepared raw. All pickles were cooked or processed by some method. They also abstained when dining out.

My take and my cousins' take on the incident was that the airway may have been blocked by a piece of the pickle; the heat was too much for her; she had a food allergy to the pickle; or the baby's system could not tolerate the raw pickle.

I have related this story to others over the years. Several people seem to think the story is funny. They say, "Gerry's aunt died eating pickles." Everyone concurs that it is tragic that she died, but the oddity provides some semblance of humor. This is part of the human equation; as long as you are not directly affected by the misfortune, you can find comedy in something out of the ordinary.

Humor can also be an outlet for being uncomfortable with a situation or attempting to disguise how a person feels down inside. The person close to the misfortune can either be hurt by the joking or can realize that no harm is intended. Teasing and gossip can have similar developments, depending on the person. That's life when you live in a jungle, and even if you don't live in a jungle, that's life.

# Piano Mom

M Y MOTHER PLAYED PIANO CONSIDERABLY well. She played songs by ear. She would listen to a song on the radio or television tinker around with it, and eventually play the song completely from memory. She could really tickle the ivories.

My sister attended piano lessons for a number of years. She played the instrument for several functions. My mother tried to coax me into taking lessons. In those days, a boy did not play piano in our locale. Playing was not considered virile. No matter how hard my mother tried to convince me to learn to play, I resisted ardently. She didn't harp on it but tried to band with my relatives to get me to take lessons. My mother and sister tried to teach me a few notes along the way, but I never advanced past plunking out a few tunes with one hand-nothing noteworthy to mention.

I purchased a guitar when I was in college. I fretted over it for awhile but couldn't master it, and I quit it calmato.

Mom basically played for her own pleasure. Very seldom did she play in any other forum but our home. My dad, as I said, never spent time in a tavern. Once in a while when he visited my aunt, his sister, and my uncle, he drank a small glass of homemade wine my uncle had made, but that was the only alcohol he consumed. My mom would have beer on a rare occasion. My uncle, who was my sponsor when I was confirmed in the Catholic church, held a gathering of my mother's family in January 1962. The get-together was eight months after my dad passed away. She had been mourning my pa's death. For whatever reason, she decided to have more than one beer.

I was in the basement with my cousins, playing cards. All of a sudden, we heard sounds of the playing of my uncle and aunt's piano and others singing. We decided to join the entertainment. When we arrived, we witnessed my mother playing the piano with a beer setting on the bridge where sheet music was intended to be placed. She was played and singing without the need for sheet music. She played and sang with the other family members for about an hour and a half. One of the songs she played was one of her favorites, "Under the Double Eagle," which was a real upbeat song for the times. I think she played that song twice.

It was the first and only time I ever saw her a bit tipsy.

I had watched classic movies and television shows where a person portrayed an individual who was not known for drinking and had a few drinks, a fortuitous movement, and became very joyous as my mother did, but watching firsthand was an enjoyable experience.

Mom always had a hearty laugh when she was enjoying herself; it would make you laugh along with her. She never needed anything to pep her up to enjoy life. My mom died in 1967, and she never again drank more than one beer on any occasion, but everyone always remembered with a smile the day my mom played and sang. I believe it was good therapy for my mom. She did have one more experience a few years later with alcohol which was more of an accidental impairment.

There is a story about God looking around heaven and finding several renowned sinners present in heaven. He goes to Saint Peter and tells him he is not doing his job. Saint Peter says, "My Lord, I am doing my job. I rejected them at the gates, but they go to the back gate, and your mother lets them in." This was the way of mothers in the days I was growing up. My mother and aunts were no exception. My mother would sometimes get so angry with me and others that she could not see straight, but she would also be very forgiving. Sometimes it was awhile before she would forgive, and sometimes it was subtle but forgiveness was always complete.

When I was little, my mom once said to my dad that adults' hands were too big to spank children. Some people have agreed that my backside should have been tanned a few times. Verbal conditioning seemed to work well for both my parents. My mother could get to the point specifically. After I grew older, the bottom of the stairs was no longer an option.

After my dad's death, when we moved from the farm to a small house in the city twelve miles southeast of our farm, I was fourteen years old. Privileges were taken away along with verbal one-way discussions from my mother. If I caused trouble in school, I received double punishment at home. Soon after, though, total forgiveness was always given.

A list of offenses was always stored in my mother's memory bank for future reference. When discussing a present misdemeanor, she would remind me, for history's sake, that I was not a model young man.

My mother had a great deal of pride. When my dad died, we basically lost our farm due to doctor and hospital bills. Therefore, the small home my mother purchased was nothing elaborate. She would not take any financial gifts or handouts.

Mom had a friend who lived in Ohio that she kept in contact with by mail. This friend was very well off. The friend had a medical condition which made it difficult for her to travel. Mom's pride overcame her. She had my sister take a picture in front of a house down the street, which was much larger than our house and had better landscaping and outbuildings. She sent the picture to her friend and noted that this was our home.

A short time later, she felt guilty that she was so vain. It also was in the back of her mind that her friend might visit someday. This never happened. My sister and I found this humorous for two reasons; first of all, watching her when she thought about what she had done; and secondly, this was so out of character for her to fudge the truth. We never let her know our impressions, though; that would have only made things worse.

My mother was a grand woman. It is true that the hand that rocks the cradle rules, making all the difference in the world of how a child matures. You can learn the most about how to continue your life after you leave your home at your mother's knee, from her direction and the example she sets in living her own life. I possess a larger shoe size than my folks', but the footsteps of life they left in the sand were much larger than I have left. This can be said for many individuals of their generation, compared to my generation and my children's.

Here I will include a tribute to my mom.

# ꟿom, You're ꞃome

Every day before the sun sets
There is one whose smiling face I still see yet.
Her voice, her laughter, her love of music to me
Are roots of life which will ever important be

She became a little buttercup
One lovely spring day
Eight other flowers paved the way
A little town named Reese is where she first supped

A move was soon in the cards
The road looked rough, rocky, and hard
The world to her looked wide and deep
When she was not in mother's arms asleep

Another small town called Beal
Soon became their home
Nevermore to roam
The German ancestors had an appeal

Youth was not kind to her for sure
Death took her mother from her
Working for her family needs
Took the place of educational seeds

At night you could hear the sighing
With the sound of her heart crying
Her work and shopping in the city
Took the place of pity

A neighbor employed a hired hand
He moved her soul
However, adult reasoning took its toll

For a few years marriage was footsteps in the sand

Still the last dance many times to start
Was saved for him
Then it became when they were apart
A happy sorrow in the wind

A trust not to be broken
Became a blessed bond not to be considered a token
Two offspring came
She sang, even though their birth caused pain

The marriage was right and strong
With love it could not go wrong
With few dark days
Came many bright ones on the way

A calm rain is good
Together with a storm
A calm man is good
When fear and excitement is the norm

When brainpower is there
Devoted love and work is shared
Errors are replaced with care
There is no love that can compare

They both died.

He-when spring had sprung
When a father and son's relationship had begun
At night you could hear the sighing
With the sound of her crying

She-with much grief
Death came like a thief
A young man can show no pain

He must cry in the rain

Her voice, her laughter, her love to me
Are roots of my life
I ever see
That cannot be divided by a knife

# Tale Fifteen

# Naughty Speech

CURLY "STOOGE" WAS IN THE courtroom in a scene famous to Stooge lovers. He was asked the line, "Do you swear-." He interrupted the person before he could complete the remaining portion of the oath request, and answered, "No, but I know the words."

I cannot remember my father ever using any dirty or cuss word in front of anyone. If he did, it would have been in German. He said something in German when things were not going right for him, but I did not understand what he was saying. In English one of his sayings when something was not going smoothly was, "If that don't skin ya, I don't know what would skin ya!"

I mentioned earlier that we put cornstalks in bundles in a field. This normally was done by cutting each individual stalk with a corn knife, then placing several stalks in a combined upward bundle, and then tying the bundle with twine. The bundle then was left to dry. We retrieved them individually throughout late fall and winter.

One year before I was old enough to partake in the process, my father decided to lighten his workload and hire a young fellow who had a machine that would cut the corn and bundle it with minimal human participation. My dad and this fellow worked together on the project, and I mainly "hung out," observing this work and helping once in awhile.

On the first day during the morning session, this young man used some foul words and told some off-color jokes. After we had lunch, my dad asked him to please refrain from this line of speech, especially around me. That afternoon not much was said between my dad and him.

The next day the young gentleman used the same type of jargon. My dad did not say anything. That night, I heard him discuss the issue with my mother. The conversation centered around whether to continue lightening my dad's load or to refuse to allow the use of the F-word.

The next day the lingo continued. Later in the afternoon, my dad approached the issue. The F-words were then used by both men, my dad's words being "fed-up, festering, forbidden, flawed, foolish, and fatal." The young man's only word was the F-word. This was my first exposure to the word, and I did not even know what it meant.

My dad fired the fellow, paid the fee for his work, and bid him farewell. The young man made a feeble attempt at asking forgiveness. My dad told him he forgave him but to forget ever coming back. This fellow was the only guy in the area who had this type of machine, so we went back to cutting corn by hand for the remaining years we farmed the land.

My mother and father tended our orchard, which was more specifically a grove of individual trees south of our home. Our grove formed a horseshoe with the fruit trees forming a border approximately one hundred by eighty feet. The inside portion was where we raised potatoes each year.

The northeast corner was made up of a strawberry patch. Three apple trees lined the southeast corner. One apple tree stood between two pear trees bordering the south end of the area. Our grapevines were perpendicular to the westernmost pear tree. The area jutted out west of the grapevines to a line of trees consisting of a cherry tree, a pear tree, and two more cherry trees. One apple tree bordered the north portion of the area, located equally between the western border and eastern border. An apple tree also existed near our house.

Dad sprayed and pruned all the trees except the tree by the house, which had seen its better days of yielding fruit. This tree bestowed a rope swing originally provided for my sister by my dad. This swing, however, was much more conservative than the playground swings at school, where you would see how much you could pump to see how high in altitude you could fly. This was often discouraged by adults if they witnessed any attempts to accomplish this. This tree and the other trees also provided fun for climbing, jumping games, and other activities such as playing cowboys. Action within the trees was kept to a minimum when the trees were blossoming and actually providing fruit.

Dad's spraying techniques were very conservative, not like some who overused DDT Those individuals lived by the theory that if the prescribed amount was good, then double or triple the amount was great and would eliminate the need for more frequent spraying. This train of thought was also employed when applying fertilizer in crop production.

This resulted in insecticides such as DDT being banned and chemical intrusion of groundwater.

Two plum trees on the northwestern end of our farm basically grew wild and yielded fruit without any care. I got to know the trees almost personally, especially the fragrance and beauty of their blossoms, which I still enjoy each spring. I really got to know the cherry trees and their texture, weak spots, and tree limbs when I was procured to act as a human scarecrow each year when the birds found the cherries to be an excellent source of food just before ripening. This deployment could last two weeks. As long as I was located in one of the cherry trees, the birds avoided the trees, but they would hover close by the area, chirping as if they were disgusted with my presence. Once in a while they would dive-bomb me, flying close to my head. My position in the tree was a combination of standing and leaning against the base of the tree, with my back as my upper-body balance and a limb of the tree as the balance for my feet. Sometimes I would spend a short time in each tree so they would not get lonely.

When the cherries were considered ripe by both my mother and father (there was sometimes considerable inspection and discussion between the two of them prior to harvesting), we would pick the cherries, and Mom would can them. My second-least-favorite job, next to mowing the lawn, was removing the pits from the cherries with a hairpin prior to processing. The job was tedious and required accuracy. Mother showed great patience, although she could not understand my lack of talent in this regard. (Mother also had similar disappointment with respect to my deficiencies in penmanship, which She had gathered awards in when she attended school.)

Mom canned all our fruit throughout the summer and fall. We had our share of canned applesauce, whole cherries for winter pies and other purposes, cherry juice, and grape juice. Pears were canned, halved and quartered.

My mom did not spare the sugar when canning fruit, since sugar was reasonably priced during the mid 1950s, even though just ten to twelve years earlier sugar was rationed during World War II. My mom said my uncle, the DeKalb salesman, said at the time of the rationing, "What are they doing over there fighting the war-throwing sugar cubes at the enemy?"

Mom made fresh fruit pies each week throughout the summer and fall. We ate fruit off the tree also, both seasons. Grapes, late apples, and pears made a nice treat after getting home from school. Strawberries were eaten in June, and Mother made jam with them. I don't recall us ever making cider. In fact, I really don't ever remember even drinking cider until we moved off the farm, and Mom bought some in a Kroger grocery store when I was a senior in high school.

We would go each year to pick blackberries with my uncle that was my sponsor and my cousins on state land in mid-August. Many times my sister, my cousins, and I ate more than we picked. The older we got, though, the more we were required to be steadfast in our picking for berries to take home.

I recall the weather being hot and humid when we picked them; we always took water with us to stay hydrated. One year my cousin who was a year younger than me threw a ladle full of water at me. Of course I had to retaliate. My father caught me in action. He raised his voice and told me to stop the fooling around. I came up with what I thought was a brilliant answer. I said that we were trying to cool each other off. My uncle said he and my dad were not going to buy that, and to get back to picking.

We would always eat a few of the berries with sugar and milk; Mom would make a couple of pies; and the remaining portions were made into jam. Apples that fell on the ground were fed to pigs which we raised for our own source of meat for a few years.

In spite of all our fruit, I can't remember seeing many deer. Deer were not plentiful in the immediate area around our farm for some reason, possibly because of cattle being present in the surrounding area. Pheasants were abundant in the grain fields when I was young, but when I was in my teens, they disappeared. Insecticides and predators were blamed for their reduction.

One day our neighbor down the road visited our farm with his son and his son's buddy. They asked my dad if they could hunt for deer on our property. They said they had seen deer on the back portion of our land. My dad said they could but told them jokingly, "My cows are back there; don't shoot one."

They were gone for about an hour and came back stone-faced, saying they had shot one of our cows. They said they would pay for the cow, but if Dad could get the tractor to pull the cow up to the barn, they would go get their truck to haul the cow to be slaughtered. Dad came to the house and told my mom in so many words that he was not happy with the man and boys; however, he did not swear or raise his voice.

The three culprits got down the road about a quarter mile and came back and said it was just a joke. The man said the boys cooked up the scheme when they got bored with hunting, and my dad's comment put the idea in their heads. (This man was known for a crazy sense of humor.) My dad said, "I should have known. I would expect something like this from your son and his friend, but a grown man should know better than to go along with it. You, being a farmer, should know how important a farmer's cows are to him, so the next time you get bored, try to do something a little more worthwhile." The man just said, "Sorry, but you must admit it was pretty funny for awhile there." Then he left with the boys. My dad later said to my mom, "That man will never change."

When I was eleven years old, the apple tree nearest to the strawberry patch was providing fewer apples, and their size had diminished. I was allowed to place a tree house in this tree. This structure provided an area for reading books and just enjoying the outdoors. I spent a number of nights sleeping in this open-air home.

# Golden Rule Days

WHEN MY UNCLE THE PLUMBER went by our house, I would run out to the road to an area west of our house. There I would wave at him, and he would smile and wave back. One morning in June 1957 when he went by our house, I did the usual action of waving, and he smiled and waved back. That afternoon my uncle who was our township supervisor, visited us. I was sent out to pick strawberries. I surmised that they were going to talk about adult matters like someone in the family being pregnant or something like that.

When my uncle was leaving, he had a grave look on his face. He came out to the strawberry patch and made some small talk with me. He acted uneasy. After he drove off, I went back in the house. I was informed that my uncle the plumber had suffered a heart attack while working in a well pit. "How is he doing?" I asked. My mom paused and said, "He did not make it," a term used by our family when someone dies. I was overwhelmed. My uncle was a special man. Most the young boys and girls knew of his special love for them. He always promised them to take them to Big Rock Candy Mountain, where there was all the candy you wanted, and every wish you ever wanted was fulfilled. He had a special method of relating to children. I guess you could say he went to his own "Rock Candy Mountain."

Three of my uncle and aunt's children were still in high school. My aunt needed to find work. She had a teaching certificate, so she was hired to teach fourth grade for the school year 1957-58. Guess who was in fourth grade that year? My aunt was my godmother. I was excited when she dropped by the house to tell me she would be my teacher. She acted excited too.

Her excitement diminished a bit as the year went on, when she discovered that I was not a young boy who avoided mischief. Although I was not too much of a rascal, we did have some moments when she needed to discipline me. She tried hard to work with me on my penmanship, but like others before her and after, she found that the battle could not be won.

My aunt's manner of discipline centered around soliciting prayer for the individual who created the discord. Having the transgressor write multiple sentences was also an option for a penalty. This choice of punishment was evidently used when my aunt was young. This task, however, did not improve my penmanship. My cousin had an artful method of using two pencils at a time to write his sentences. He said it cut his time spent in half. I tried it once, but it seemed to be more of a burden, and one pencil was enough of a challenge for me anyway. My aunt seemed to understand very well the stages of development in a young person's life, evidently from raising three boys and five girls.

The final hour and final day of my fourth year in elementary school was spent in the fifth grade classroom. Sister B was the fifth grade teacher. She made a speech about her discipline techniques and pointed out a paddle she had hanging by one of the blackboards in the room. A few of her students were asked to verify her statements, and they confirmed them. Even though this was the first we had heard of her hard-shelled attitude, many of us sure as sugar believed her. I was beside myself on the ride home on the bus. My first objective when I arrived home was to rush to talk to my dad. My dad was on our tractor trimming some weeds with our hay mower, on the outer edges of our cornfield. I stopped him, and he slid over on the seat so I could sit on the seat with him. I began to discuss the future school year with him. In his usual calming manner, he told me it would not be as bad as I thought. This appeased me for a while, but throughout the summer it was still on my mind. The closer the time came to begin school the more concerned I became regarding my welfare.

The first day arrived. The bus ride to school was too short. When my classmates and I entered the room, there was my aunt. She was going to team-teach with another teacher for our class until Sister B returned from having surgery on her knee that summer. She was not going to return until mid-October.

Then sometime in the first week in October, it was announced that Sister B was coming back the next day. She was coming back sooner than originally thought. I was nerved up again.

The next day arrived and to our surprise, Sister B was rather mild mannered. When we were released for recess, the topic of our discussion was how she had apparently changed. We reasoned that it was because of her surgery.

As time went by, we learned that this was Sister B's normal demeanor. We learned that she liked to play jokes on others. We discovered that the presentation on the last day of school the previous year was only an act in a so-called play, and she and the class were the players in the show. When Sister B spoke, you listened. But she was a wonderful person and not mean at all. I don't recall the paddle ever leaving its designated area. Sister B was, in fact, one of my favorite teachers.

Several of my classmates and I developed a habit of sticking our fingers in our shoes and pulling on the shoe when attempting to answer a question. Sister B would always say, "Stop playing with your toe jam and keep your fingers out of your shoes and answer the question."

All desks in those days had an opening which at one time was used for an ink bottle. Ink pens in years past were manually filled by placing the pen in the ink bottle, then manipulating a lever and filling the pen with ink. These openings were called ink wells. Pencils and ballpoint pens replaced these units for recording information. My sister related that these pens were untidy to work with, and you could stain your clothes if you were not careful. She also said the pens were a source of mischief for boys. If you pulled the lever forward after filling it, you could use the pen similar to a squirt gun and spray a victim.

Sister B told us to store our "toe jam" in these openings. She told us that the toe jam would turn into something she called and pronounced "too-mos-see". She called the openings too-mos-see holes. She said the janitor would clean the hole at the end of each week. She had other quirks she introduced to us for fun. We realized these were rather silly, but we had fun just the same.

One day Sister B left the room and left one of my classmates in charge. Sister B told this classmate to write down on the blackboard anybody that talked or misbehaved. Soon after she left, a boy who could best be described as a "real character" began throwing paper wads. The monitor wrote his name down on the blackboard in front of the room. The character told him, since he could write so well, to write his name down again, which he did. We had three blackboards in front of the room and two lining the west end of the room. The two pupils continued the daring and writing until the recorder had written the gentleman's name across every blackboard in the room.

When Sister B returned, she asked what possessed the recorder, and what was the purpose of the writing across the boards. The boy stood mute. Sister B said, "I tell you what happened, class; two boys got carried away with foolishness. Foolishness can be funny in its place, but this foolishness is out of place, and this is a result of two young men trying to show off for their classmates." The boys never received punishments. She told us we should all learn from the experience. However, I don't recall that those of us who were prone to goofing off slowed down much when we wanted to get into mischief. When we grew older, we all agreed that Sister B was right and was trying to influence us to shape up.

We had two incidents involving noses during Sister B's tenure with our class. One involved the boy who was the front end of the camel for the "Three Kings" with me. We attended lunch in the basement of the church. The outer entrance to the cafeteria was not heated and had less-than-ideal steps down to the basement. The boys always rushed to be first in line to eat. Shoving each other was not out of the question on the way to our destination. On this given day, we were all shoving each other going down the steps. This was not unusual, as I said. The aforementioned boy went rolling face-first down the steps. His folks were called to take him to the doctor. About two hours later, his mother returned with him. Sister B and his mother made him go around the room for our class to observe his nose while he lifted the bandage for us to see what happens when you mess around.

Sister B tried to get the boy to tell on who pushed him. He never told on the culprits, but about four or five boys had a hand in it, so to speak,- yours truly being one who could have been fingered. We stopped pushing and shoving for the remaining portion of the year, because there was always an adult monitoring our action, making certain that we walked single file (the proper method of walking together as a group which is appropriate even today). The boy was left with a small indentation in his nose.

The other incident occurred when my classmates and I were playing baseball. One of my classmates was batting. I knew he often threw his bat. Another classmate was standing nearby. I moved to tell him to step back. Just as I was warning him, the bat flew out of the hitter's hands and landed square on my nose. I began bleeding. Some of my classmates ran to get Sister B. By the time she arrived, the bleeding had subsided a bit. Sister B told me, basically, to suck it up and get over it. I felt she could have had a little more compassion. My classmate who threw the bat was not told to stop throwing the bat, but I was told to watch out next time.

It stuck in my craw for a few days that she did not feel some sympathy for me. I approached the issue with her one day. She said, "You have to learn to be tough. I saw that you were not in danger. I surmised that you only had a nosebleed. It bothered me more than you thought, but I need to teach you boys and girls that life can have ups and downs, and you need to deal with them." She said further that she would discuss the issue of throwing the bat with all my classmates. I was satisfied.

When I look back on my time with Sister B, I feel we learned the basics of life from her, along with being educated through school subjects. She was fair, and if you needed an explanation for one of her actions, she tried to answer you without making you feel inferior. She was always approachable to talk to about your concerns in life. She also could read you when you were having a rough time. She would try to comfort you.

We went through the same ritual at the end of the year, bringing in the students from fourth grade. We rehearsed our parts along with her. We did not sell it well, because this grade had been clued in, in advance, to some degree prior to the presentation.

Sister B did not return the next year, so the scam was unneeded. Later on in life, I learned Sister B was a "tomboy" when she was young.

I have never had the fortune to have someone appear to me in a dream or under any other circumstances. I have, though, experienced some oddities in my life.

I was caught lighting matches by my mother when I was seven years old. She had gone to the chicken coop to gather eggs. I decided to try to light a torch like configuration made up of pages from a magazine. My mother decided to check her flower beds and arrive in the house through a door we seldom used on our front porch. As she approached the door, she saw me through the window of the door. The pitfalls of this action were discussed in great detail.

When my oldest daughter was eight years old, I caught her lighting toilet paper in a similar manner. I had just finished mowing the lawn and approached the door that went into our living room from the front porch. I observed her in the action of lighting the paper through the window of that door. We sat down and had a chat similar to the one I had had with my mother.

My grandson came up to visit us for a few weeks from his home near Ann Arbor, Michigan. Soon after he arrived, we smelled the odor of sulfur;

then we found remnants of a few burned matches in drawers. Since no one smoked in the house, my wife and I approached our grandson. After some denial, he admitted to the offense. A discussion was again held regarding the risks.

When my oldest was going into fourth grade, she had never had a male teacher. On the last day of third grade, her class was guided into the fourth grade room to meet their teacher. Their teacher was a male, and he described his discipline in detail, which included a paddle which hung in the classroom.

Yogi Berra's "déjà vu all over again" came into play.

My daughter came home with tears streaming down her face. I just happened to have the day off from work. I related the story about my discussion with my dad years earlier and the results. She said she heard from others who were in his classroom that he actually used the paddle on kids. I told her if this was so, she did not have anything to worry about, because she never caused problems. I think she still had her doubts after our discussion, though, and continued to have them throughout the summer.

After the first day of school, she came home to say, "You were right, Dad! He is just like you. He tells jokes and sings. We had fun singing, and he told some jokes." I don't recall my daughter ever coming home and saying he used the paddle.

One day when I was playing golf with her teacher years later, the topic came up. Her teacher said if he would have used the paddle, my daughter would never have had to worry, as she was a model student.

# TALE SEVENTEEN

## Big Sister

M Y SISTER AND I USUALLY enjoyed each other's company when she was about twelve and I was about six. One deed we did together was killing gophers that invaded our lawn. My dad engaged my sister and I to rid the premises of these rodents. We would run water in the hole with a hose at one end and wait at the other end with a baseball bat for the gopher to escape his waterlogged home. I normally manned the execution area, as I had a little quicker reaction with the weapon of choice.

Sometimes this was a hit-and-miss proposition. If we missed, we would need to wait a couple hours for the hole to clear of water. It amazed us that the critters would return to the hole after the traumatic experience of us flooding the hole and swinging a weapon at them. Although as I remember it, if the gopher managed to escape our wrath, the beast would try to withstand the water longer and would become weakened to a point that it was easier to institute capital punishment.

We eventually eliminated all the vermin from our lawn. In later years my dog Fido, who entered my life when I was nine, became adept at bagging these unwanted excavators.

The second task we tackled together was trying to nurse two sick calves. My dad always had good luck with not losing a calf. This pattern rang true before and after 1954. The year 1954 brought two newborn calves from two different cows. The poor offspring had problems with normal stools and could not retain milk nursed from their mother. Finally, they would not nurse. My dad gave my sister and me the job of bottle-feeding a combination of milk and medicines to the two patients. They were both female calves, so Dad told us that if we could save them, he would keep them instead of taking them to the weekly auction. Normally after calves had reached four to five months old, they were taken to the auction to be sold. The actual time to take them depended on what the demand on futures of calves was.

One calf was the normal black and white colors; the other had red and white coloring. We fed them three times a day and spent time watching their progress. At first the black and white one appeared to improve, and the red and white one seemed to be losing ground. After about a week, they changed conditions. The red and white calf became stronger, and the other one started going downhill. I believe it was about the eleventh or twelfth day when the black and white one died.

The red and white one improved each day. As could be expected, we had mixed emotions. Burying the other calf was sad, but we put all our happy emotions into the red and white one. The calf grew into a heifer and thereafter into a cow. We called her Reddy. In 1958, Dad kept another calf that was almost all white. The Hanna-Barbera cartoon Ruff and Reddy became popular in 1957, so I wanted to call this new cow Ruff. I lost out to Snow White, my dad and mom's choice. Reddy was beloved by the whole family because of the miracle of life. Plus she did yield more milk than the other cows most of the time. It was difficult to sell her after Dad died, but two brothers who farm together bought her and took good care of her. I visited her and Barney and Doll a few times.

Although I tried to avoid picking my nose, my sister and I did pick wildflowers together each spring. Our woods provided a variety of flowers from violets to a flower we called Sweet Williams. Once a week from the last week in April to the last week in May, we would walk back to our wooded area to collect these items of beauty. The edge of the timber was the best location. My mother would accompany us once per year. In fact, when we were old enough to walk, she brought my sister and I to the woods to pick flowers. She required that you become acquainted with gathering flowers, like a father who enjoys sports requires his sons and daughters to learn to be an athlete. A bucket which had special partitions in it to separate each bouquet, was brought to the location.

My sister and I really enjoyed going through this process together. Part of any trip to the woods was to visit a huge oak tree. This tree was very tall, and its circumference was extensive. No trip was made without my sister and I extending our arms around the tree, trying to touch fingers. We hoped as we grew older that our arms would lengthen to a point that we could touch fingers, although my mom and dad as adults could not do so. This ritual was similar to that of a boy or girl trying to touch higher points by jumping or standing flat-footed as they grow. This measure of progress in height has been an action of each youth from one generation to another. Dad sold the tree and some others to a company. Although he made money selling the timber, it was a sad day just the same, to see it being cut down.

Playing nun, which consisted of dressing in habits my mother made for us, was another event which we performed together. Attendance at Catholic ceremonies was the method of our play. An altar was set up in my sister's bedroom for this objective. We used Necco Wafers to receive communion.

Another room was set up with desks that had been retrieved by my dad from an old, one-room schoolhouse that had been torn down across the road in 1943. Imaginary students were available to be taught by my sister. I was the nun who was responsible for playground supervision and the distribution of library books. I also played dolls with my sister, paper dolls, and regular dolls.

I participated in many feminine pastimes with my sister over the years. When I told my male friends about my childhood bonding with my sister, I received some disparaging remarks. I, however, did not or still do not have any concerns with my masculinity.

My sister did have a few dupes she pulled on me. The harshest was when she told me, when I was four, that chicken hawks could swoop down and carry off little kids my weight. She told me to run for cover when I saw one hovering around. She told me that it was my responsibility to do this; she said my folks did not have time to watch out for me. For some reason, I did not check with my parents to verify this information. This went on for about a month until one day we were walking along, and a hawk began circling our yard. My sister yelled, "Run, boy, run!" I quickly ran for the house. My mother was in the kitchen developing bread. She questioned the scared look on my face. When I explained, my sister was summoned. She told my mother it was just a joke. My sister was told to tell me she was sorry. Mother said she did not have time for an immediate punishment, because she needed to complete her work. Either my mother forgot, or my sister's record of not getting into trouble caused no further desire in my mom's mind for correction. A few days later, I asked my sister whether she had experienced any further discussion regarding her efforts to trick me. She said she did not have any such deliberation, and I better not bring the subject up again. When I informed her I might just do that, she stuck out her tongue at me and tilted her head from side to side. I, of course, knew better than to test the waters in this regard, since my sister had been a member of the family longer than I had. I was still in training, and she was my big sister.

As we grew older, the six years between us in age caused more of a rift between us. Even when we were younger, my sister needed her space. Therefore when her little brother commented on something, many times it went on deaf ears.

It was a few days before Christmas 1950. I had just turned three years old on December 12. My folks went Christmas shopping while my sister was in school. I accompanied them. They bought a substantial amount of candy. On the way home, since I had been a good boy while they were shopping, they decided to give me a few pieces of the candy to snack on. I was exposed to the larger quantity when they retrieved the pieces.

My sister had given up candy for Advent, which was customary for a Catholic child to do in those days more times than not. Evidently they felt because I had been treated to the candy, she should be allowed a one-day reprieve from the abstinence. A few pieces were placed in a bowl for her to snack on when she arrived home from school.

When she arrived home, she saw the treat on the living room table. She excitedly said, "Ooh, candy!" To which I said, "There's 'yots' more than that yet." Ignoring my comment, my sister began to eat a piece of candy. I again repeated, "There's yots more than that yet." It is my understanding, from having this story related to me by all involved, that I continued this effort a few more times. However, my sister approached the issue somewhere between believing that I was enjoying going on about nothing and the thought pattern of W.C. Fields: "Go away kid, you bother me."

My mother fearing that if I continued too long, my sister would catch on, told me to go play in the kitchen with my toys. I soon became concerned with other projects.

# Dogs I Have Known

GROUCHO MARX ONCE SAID, "OUTSIDE of a dog a book is a man's best friend. Inside of a dog it's too dark to read." Charles Schultz said, "As soon as a child is born, he should be issued a dog."

I danced with three ugly girls one night; it was a "Three Dog Night."

In my lifetime, nine dogs have entered my life. The first I already mentioned; the St. Bernard that my godfather gave me was not a good starter dog. I was too young for such a large dog, and he was an outlaw who killed chickens and was a dirty, egg-sucking dog.

My second dog was a keeper. He entered my life when I was nine years old. He was one of a litter of eight. He was the only one who amounted to anything. The rest were bums. My uncle who was our township supervisor owned the mother, and the father was unknown. We always said he was like his mother, and the others must have been like the father. The owners of the other dogs soon gave up on them. I named him Fido. His mother was a collie. He was my buddy.

When he was about six months old, I visited the barn to get some milk for him from one of our cows. He followed me into the barn. He began barking at a calf which was about three weeks old. As I led the cows in the barn to place them in their stanchions, the mother of the calf was evidently distraught that Fido was barking at the calf. She went ballistic and slammed me against the barn wall. Although she had been dehorned, she caught me with the stub of her horn. I passed out for a short period of time. When I came to, Fido was hovering over me, protecting me from the cow. I had a lump on my head from hitting the cement wall and had a cut on my stomach.

I managed to get my bearings to put the cows in their stanchions. Fido guarded me from any further assault by the cow in question. Crying was not allowed at my age. I ran up to our house and received treatment from my mother for my wounds. My dad was surprised when he heard of that particular cow attacking me. His surprise was because this cow always had problems birthing a calf. In fact, this cow was how I received my orientation regarding how a calf really came into the world, when I helped my mother pull a calf manually from the mother. This occurred when my dad was in the hospital before he died. After she birthed an offspring, she basically rejected the product. She would not allow it to nurse. So it was unusual for her to be skittish about her calf's welfare.

Fido would sometimes be sent to gather the cows from the pasture. He would really be gentle when he rounded up the cattle. This pleased my dad. If you rushed the cattle, my dad felt their milk production would be affected. Fido once in awhile would nip at the legs of the cow who hurt me. He was gentle, but he was also protective. He drove off a few solicitors in his time. He seemed to know the difference between friend and foe.

Fido could hang by himself, discovering new adventures or building on old ones. When it came time to spend time with me, he was always ready to go on a quest for fun. He was always at my side. We would go on walks together and play games of fetch.

My mother was not fond of dogs. Fido seemed to know this, as he would follow at a short distance behind her, trying not to get in the way but making sure she knew he was with her. He would perform a little dance, jumping on his back feet and circling around her whenever she spent time outdoors. His favorite thing to do was to follow her to the door of the chicken house when she visited the structure to gather eggs. She would pet him when they ended their journey.

My dad would talk to him, but Fido seemed to know he was busy and would keep his distance. My sister had a dog when she was five or six who was hit by a car and died. For this reason, she said she did not want to get close to Fido and, after all, he was my dog.

I would sing to him, "Can you speak nice, little Fido, can you speak nice?" He would bark while I sang to him. We would go on for a while doing this. He also shook hands with anyone who asked him to. He had a knack for killing skunks without getting sprayed. Every once in awhile we would see a dead skunk he had eradicated in the yard. At the time we moved off the farm into the city, Fido must have gotten into a fight with another critter, as he was torn up badly. For this reason and because my mom thought he would not be happy in town, he was left behind. It was hard leaving him.

About two weeks after we were settled in our house in the city, Mom asked my sister and me to take two washtubs and visit the farm to obtain some richer soil for a garden she wanted to plant. (We called them washtubs because we gathered rainwater in them to wash our hair with. My parents thought in those days that washing your hair with rainwater gave the hair a good texture.)

When we arrived, Fido came running. He was all healed. I wanted to bring him with us, but my sister tried to convince me this would upset my mother. My love for Fido got the better of me. I talked him into getting in the car. We arrived back at our house in town. My plan was to leave Fido in the car until I could soften up my mom. However, Fido had other ideas. He jumped out too quick for me as I opened the door and ran to my mother, who was out in the backyard. Mother was surprised at first of course, then she smiled. Without any objection, she said, "Well okay, you can have him here, but get him a structure to house him in." I built him a doghouse and bought a chain to keep him in our yard. He was located next to our house.

I would let Fido loose when I was home so I could play with him, but we feared that he might not stay in the yard. Therefore, when I was not with him we kept him tied. We still had a great deal of fun together, but I had less time to spend with him, as I became busier with school functions. This program lasted for two years. Then one day my mother told me he had to be moved to the back of our property near the alley. She did not like the odor by the house, and he began to damage the siding with his chain.

At first, it was okay, then some kids began throwing stones at him when they walked by. This understandably upset him. One day one of these kids moved too close when throwing a stone, and Fido bit him. The kid's mother was upset. I tried to make a plea for Fido's case but my mother would not have any of it. Two days later we called the dog warden. When he came to pick him up, he said, "You're going to have to give that dog to me. Why? I watched that dog for two years; now he is a wonderful dog." I explained the circumstances, and when he went to take him, he snapped at him. He was surprised, but he said, "Well, that's what happens when a dog is mistreated."

He said he would try to find a home for him back out in the country where he could run free. However, I knew it was probably a trip to the death chamber for him. It was a sad ending for a wonderful scout.

My third dog was a dachshund. Our neighbor in the mobile home park we lived in the second year my wife and I were married was given two puppies by her mother-in-law. They talked me into taking one of the puppies. I was going to college, my wife was working, and our first child was about six months old. The dog's name was Arthur. I thought a dog of German descent might be good to have and would be well disciplined. Wiener dogs were also fashionable. My wife had about the same fondness for dogs as my mother. The combination of my wife's position regarding dogs, Arthur not taking to my daughter, his habit of chewing on anything and everything, and the lack of time to spend with him provided guidance for giving him his walking papers. A family several mobile homes away from ours took Arthur after he had spent three months in our home. We moved away from the park a year later, so I do not know the final results of that relationship. However, although it was not heaven for them, it appeared to be an acceptable kinship from my observation.

About a year later we were again talked into taking in a poor waif. She had already had six owners. She was a cross between a schnauzer and a poodle. She had been mistreated by her first owner, and each owner thereafter felt sorry for the dog but had to give her up for one reason or another. This dog bonded very well with my daughter but would not stay home. She would leave for a week and then come back. She had been "fixed", so I did not know the reason for her travels.

One day, she decided to chew on a plug from a lamp. This put her into shock, literally. We called the vet. He said to just let her alone for a few hours, and she would get better. We isolated her in our bedroom. She did indeed come out of it; however, after that she was not as cordial to my daughter. Since she ran away periodically and no longer was a good companion for my daughter, off she went to a new home. A friend of my wife's cousin took her. One day she ran out to the road and was run over by a car. Her name was Nickey, but Unlucky would have been a better name.

The fifth was a German shepherd, another female. My oldest daughter had surgery on her eyes when she was five years old to correct a muscle problem. The year was 1975. She was blind for a few days after the surgery. When her eyesight returned and she returned home, she asked me if she could have a dog. She said she wanted a German shepherd to protect her from a Saint Bernard who lived in our mobile home park. The Saint

Bernard always knocked her down, and she wanted some paybacks. We went to the nearest animal control and found a six-month-old shepherd. My daughter named her Shanty.

From the first day she entered our life, she barked no matter where she spent her time. She was like a newborn baby, wanting to be fed constantly. We moved to this park in 1973 when I obtained a job working for a health department in its Environmental Protection Division. We held off getting a dog because of our past experiences with having a dog in a mobile home park. Again our problems came knocking. Complaints began to multiply each day regarding the continued barking. Plus, my lack of sleep began to influence my work.

The owner of the park informed me one day that Shanty was barking up the wrong tree and had to go. My daughter had mixed emotions regarding the shepherd; she liked her, but the dog was even getting on her young nerves. After two months of ownership, the dog was given to nice couple who lived on a farm five miles out of town. After three experiences with dogs in mobile home parks, we became dog-tired, so to speak.

Snoopy: "Never waste time barking if you don't have anything to say."

The spring of 1977, our mobile home was getting too small for our three children and their parents. We found a home to rent three blocks from the public school, purchasing the home a year later. We placed our mobile home up for sale. An older lady who was getting a divorce purchased the unit. Along with the payment, we received a dresser, a king-sized bed, and a two-month-old beagle puppy. The beagle became known as Joey. Joey was born in a barn, so the outdoors was his preference. My wife found this to her liking, because she always thought dogs belonged in the area of open spaces. The great outdoors became his favorite world.

I always placed a generous amount of straw in his doghouse for fall and winter seasons and added as needed. The winter of 1978 had terribly cold weather for an extended period of time. One night when it was five below zero, I coaxed Joey into our back room for protection from the elements. He tore up our linoleum floor in protest because he was unhappy.

Joey was a wonderful dog. He had a real personality. He had a way of cocking his head when he wanted attention. He also was ready for action, though, and enjoyed any activity my kids and I could provide. He especially enjoyed my oldest daughter. You could tie him up or let him run free in the yard; he would not leave the yard.

Because we lived close to the school and other businesses, several people walked by our house each day. These individuals could walk by without concerning Joey, but the minute they stepped foot on our property, off the sidewalk, he protested. If any meter reader or such person tread in his territory, he let them know he was present. Most of the time, we had to make certain he was tied up because he would cause fear to the poor souls. Joey would not harm the person, but he would raise enough upheaval to scare people off and protect us.

In the spring of 1982, some kids decided to challenge Joey by throwing items at him when he was near the sidewalk. As a result, he started drifting away from our property. One night we received a telephone call that he was down at a nearby gas station cornering individuals. I had been working in our garage and let him loose to run about our yard. I had gotten busy and lost track of him.

When I came to pick him up, he hung his head. However, the drifting continued. Finally, to avoid problems similar to what occurred with Fido, we found a restaurant owner in the area who liked to hunt, so he took him. They developed an excellent friendship, and the owner said Joey was a good working dog. Unfortunately, Joey developed cancer three years later and died. I never told my three daughters until several years after his death.

We went a few years without a dog. Fish and parakeets were the pets of choice. We buried four parakeets and three fish in our backyard between 1982 and 1988. My youngest daughter and middle daughter bought separate parakeets in 1986. The night after the purchase was made our middle daughter's bird was found dead. We took it back, and after some tribulation regarding accusations of our assassination of the bird, we were given another. The replacement, Kirby, lived with the original Widget for two years, but he was bullied by Widget constantly. We always blamed Widget for killing his first partner. Kirby always looked helpless, and his feathers were always shaggy, but he seemed to survive and stay clear when Widget decided to become aggressive.

One night I decided to let Kirby out of his cage like I had before to give him some relief from Widget. He flew around and landed on my shoulder a few times and stayed for a bit. After a couple hours, I lost track of him because I became interested in a movie on television. I looked down at the corner of the couch near the leg. Just as I was about to say to my wife, "What is that on the floor?" I realized it was Kirby. We all said the standard, "He probably is in a better place." This is something that is not found acceptable as a response to death today. We buried him in the backyard.

Widget did not seem to be in mourning. In face, he seemed delighted. He sang and chirped loudly from that day forward. He would make so much noise that people who would call on the telephone would think we had a house full of birds.

My wife always had the job of cleaning the cage for the birds, along with the fish tank. Widget required the use of a glove to remove him from the cage, as he would bite. The removal and replacement was my job. I believe it was 1993 when my wife decided enough was enough with cleaning the cage. Living with "Lotta Noise" finally was too much for her. We gave him to a young lady who lived alone. Over the next couple of months when we called her to see how he was doing, we could hear him in the background. She left town two years later, and he was still alive. The life span of our other parakeets was three to four years. This was considered a normal life span by all those in the bird world. Widget was nine years old and still going. As far as I know, he could still be alive.

A friend of mine who was divorced three times said it sounded like maybe Widget was a female, since she enjoyed living alone and making other people miserable. I, of course, did not agree. Enough said about that. Being married for over forty years, I learned a long time ago to watch what I agreed with, at least in front of my wife.

In 1988, another dog entered our life. Out of the blue, a lady friend of my wife and I approached us about two dogs she rescued from an owner who was abusing them. A mother and her son were the two sorry creatures. My friend said she could keep the mother, but she needed a home for the son. They were basset hounds. The dog's name was Duke, and he was about two years old.

Duke was probably the dumbest and stubbornest dog that I ever met. If you told him not to do something, he peed. If you talked to him nice, he peed. We took him to the vet. She could not find anything wrong with him. He would run and be gone for two or three days. I had him neutered, and he just seemed more stupid. I tried to teach him to stay, but just when I thought I was making progress, he would run and be gone for awhile.

We would hear from people that they had seen him, but he would run when they tried to capture him. He would then come home eventually. When he was home, he was lazier than all get-out until he had a chance to run. Then he was fast-moving. When he was in the house, it would take him five minutes to walk twenty feet. He'd get up a little, move a few feet, and lay down. Some days he acted so dumb you had to point out where his food dish was, and he still had difficulty finding it. He chewed on one of my shoes at Christmas time. I yelled at him, and he went over and peed on the Christmas tree and presents in the living room. This he managed to do quickly. He was kept out of the living room until after Christmas.

The dog warden picked him up three times. He always ran to them. He must have liked jail. After a year of his fun and games and his fourth jail visit, I gave up on him. Animal control worked closely with me regarding the control of rabies. I told the officer that I was done with Sir Duke. A few days later, the officer informed me that he found a home for him with a family with two kids who could give him plenty of attention. I was not going to bet the bank on them finding true love with him.

In August 1989, I left my position as Director of Environmental Health. I took a position at another health department that was thirty-seven miles from our residence. I did not move our family for many reasons, but the main two were, first, because I did not want to move my two daughters, who were middle-school age, to another school. Secondly, we liked the area we lived in and our friends. I moved when I was my daughters' ages, and it was not a good transition at that age. It is difficult to make new friends and to be exposed to a new environment.

A need for another dog was not in anyone's cards in our family. Everyone had their priorities in place. In the spring of 1993, a gentleman who lived around the corner from us was getting divorced. He had a cocker spaniel for sale. I had always wanted a cocker spaniel. They always appeared to be neat looking and well behaved. I had also heard good things about them.

The dog owner told me he had certification the dog was registered as a purebred. He said his soon-to-be ex-wife had the papers, and he would get them for me. His name was Roscoe (the dog, not the man). I paid $150 for him, which I thought was a good price for a dog with papers.

My oldest daughter had married, and my other two daughters were in high school. My middle daughter was completing her senior year, and my youngest was at the end of her sophomore year. My youngest said, "You're on your own with this one, Dad. No one has any intentions of collaborating on taking care of a dog."

Their involvement had been limited in the past regarding care of pets. My wife had also not changed her interest in pets, and we had just removed Widget from our home. Roscoe, therefore, was my project. I built a fenced-in run approximately four feet wide and twenty feet long. I built a doghouse, which was placed at one end of the run, and placed a wooden gate at the other end of the run. I built a brick patio in front of the doghouse. I built an overhang for Roscoe, allowing him to be out of the doghouse but be protected from the heat and rain.

He did not like the inside of the house and would sit and bark if you did not play with him constantly. He would stand outside and bark constantly. He would stand in the rain and whine rather than be in protected areas. I bought him toys to play with in his run, and he would ignore them. I visited his previous owner several times during the month after I purchased him. He kept telling me he was working on getting Roscoe's papers. Then one day he went to parts unknown.

The more I got to know Roscoe, the more I began to realize he was probably not a purebred cocker spaniel. I was told a few weeks after I purchased him that cocker spaniels needed a great deal of attention. He did not just need attention; he needed a nursemaid. Plus, he gave Duke a run for his money as a thickheaded blockhead. If you threw a toy for him to retrieve, he would sit and look at you. If you had it in your hand, he pulled on it. If you let go of it, he let it sit on the floor and stared at it. It always appeared that the light was on in his head, but no one was home.

At the time, he made you feel Duke was Lassie compared to him. He would lay in the doorway of the house until you made him move, and then he would gnaw at you while you moved his sorry butt. After four months, I had had enough, and my wife found a woman from her work to take him who had three young children. They had a female Newfoundland. They lived about a mile from our house. About six months after he left our home, one morning the woman told me that Roscoe got hit by a car and did not survive. Before he left this world, he managed to get the Newfoundland pregnant with a litter. How he managed to perform this act was a mystery to everyone.

A few months later, the woman divorced her husband and moved into our neighborhood with the Newfoundland and one of Roscoe's offspring. He was a strange-looking critter. He had a thick fur pelt, and he stood rather high in stature. He had one trait of Roscoe's--he barked constantly. I guess my wife and I were lucky. Two out of three of his owners obtained a divorce.

Our youngest daughter had graduated from high school in June 1995 and was off to college, sharing an off-campus apartment with our middle daughter and two other girls. In February of 1996, empty nest syndrome was setting in. Although Roscoe had just about been the last straw regarding having a dog on our premises, I began to start searching for a dog.

A woman I worked with had three Border collies, and she tried to talk me into taking a two-year-old collie. A friend of hers was attempting to find a good home for it. I convinced my wife on a Saturday afternoon to go visit the home and the dog. She pretty much turned up her nose at the idea of letting this animal into our home. In addition, the owner indicated that she would be visiting our home periodically to make sure we were following her high standards for caring for the dog.

I remained hopeful that I would find a good dog, but I wanted to take my time, and I used different methods to search for the dog of my choice. I searched throughout the remaining portion of February, then March, and April of 1996.

Late in April of 1996, I saw an advertisement in the paper for a beagle for sale. A beagle…maybe I could get lucky with a beagle again. Joey had been a good dog.

After a great deal of coaxing, I talked my wife into visiting the home where the beagle resided. When we arrived, a gangling young man ushered us to a large pen covered with chicken wire. The beagle was housed in the pen with three Rottweilers. He was a skinny little guy. It looked like his food supply was limited to what the other dogs left for him, if… The gangling fellow and his wife raised Rottweilers. The beagle was orphaned by the man's sister who had been forced to give him up because the mobile home park they lived in did not allow dogs.

The young man let him out of his pen, and he ran around, sniffing the ground. There was something special about him that struck me. He named was Floyd, and he was registered; the papers were available and everything. He was born April 2, 1995. The gentleman wanted $100 for him. I told him my wife and I would think about it. I had already made up my mind. The "thinking about it" was convincing my wife that Floyd should enter our life. This did not go well. Our marriage vows were tested. Finally, she gave in.

We picked him up on April 29, 1996. We found out that Floyd had one problem. He had some problems traveling longer distances. When we exited the property, we didn't return home immediately; we went to the nearest Walmart, twenty miles away, to get some necessary items to raise this new member of the family.

When we reached our destination, I stayed in the truck with Floyd, and my wife purchased the items. Floyd did not look well; his head was dropping, and he could barely sit up. I kept the window open so he could breathe better. The ride home was difficult for Floyd. My wife sat next to me, and Floyd sat by the window. My wife had not sat close to me since our first year of marriage; however, romance was not in the air, since she was still a bit uninterested in sharing our happy home with this critter.

Once we arrived home, Floyd perked up. My wife had one requirement which rang true with every dog we had: no dog was allowed on the furniture at any time.

I managed to police Floyd from having any contact with the furniture all night until we were getting ready to turn in for the night. My wife was going past the living room and there sat Floyd, proud as a peacock on the top portion of the back of our couch. This caused Floyd to be placed in the backroom after I had a discussion with him on getting off on the wrong foot and how he needed to be especially good because I wanted my wife to like him. He seemed to understand.

After that, if he got on the furniture he was a little more discreet. Once or twice we caught him on the bed when we came home, but he hopped right off when we approached him. A few other times my rocker/recliner was in movement when we came home, showing evidence that he had been in it prior to our entrance.

Unlike Joey, Floyd liked to be in the house. I set up a thirty-foot leash/rope with a similar unit that stretched the length of the outer portion of our garage. This allowed Floyd to run a good portion of our property. Floyd was placed on this during the day when we were at work. He stayed in the house when we were home or gone at night.

Floyd was licensed in another county. I checked with our county regarding this, and they said he was okay until his license expired. One fine Friday in October, I came home from work to find that Floyd had slipped his collar. He was nowhere to be seen. After several hours of searching, someone informed us that the dog warden had picked him up in front of our house. The shelter was closed, so I could not bail him out. I had to wait until Monday.

Monday morning, I visited the shelter. They said since he had no identification and license (this was on his collar), they had no choice but to incarcerate him. They took me back to the cage where he was sharing a cell with other dogs. He would not look at me. I showed the warden the license tag from the other county. He said I needed one from our county. After some further discussion regarding my past discussion with our county clerk, I had to pay the fines to get him out of jail with orders to obtain another license.

On the way home, Floyd sat with his back to me. I discussed with him the money he had cost me, but he would not have any part of it. I tried to speak kindly to him, but this fell on deaf ears. When we arrived home, he went into our bedroom and would only come out to eat. He pouted for two days. He finally came out, and I guess he forgave me for his jail time.

After that we decided to have a trial period of keeping him inside while we were at work. To our surprise, Floyd never got into trouble or messed in the house. He just hung out.

Floyd was even-tempered and very seldom got too excited about anything.

We have a cemetery bordering our back property line. The last burials noted are in the 1920s, and some of the tombstones record burials in the 1840s. There is no need for a fence, because people are not dying to get in. We have awfully silent neighbors; therefore, most of the time it is rather dead around there.

The only time there is much action around there is on Memorial Day when a honor function is held each year. We have also had some fun with kids at Halloween from time to time, startling them and performing various acts of ghost skullduggery. Floyd used the cemetery as well as our backyard for running and sniffing. He loved to circle around and for you to try to catch him. There is a riverbed behind the cemetery. This was sometimes an area where Floyd drifted if his nose led him there. Retrieving him from this area took a bit of coaxing. He was like a child who is reluctant to come in from play or to go to bed at night. However, after raising my voice a few times in a demanding manner, he would give up his investigations and come running to me, and we would return to inside the house, where we would play with his toys or just enjoy each other's company.

Romping was about the extent of Floyd's excitement until a visitor came to our house. He would always greet them with a wag of his tail. He would perform a little dance, never jumping on them but always making them feel like they were welcome. He'd spend a little time with them if they wished to pet him, then adjourn back to his bed in the bedroom or to the large pillow he comforted himself with on our living room floor. If he was called upon to have bonding, he would quickly come to attention to have the interaction. Floyd loved everyone, and everyone loved Floyd. People who did not like dogs or preferred cats loved Floyd.

His disposition, as I said, was very calm. However, he would let you know when he did not like something. Someone gave me a Michigan State University blanket. I am not a fan of this sports team, so I gave it to Floyd. When he did not like something or he did not get fed when he thought it was time, he would drag his blanket out, of the bedroom to a location where we could observe it readily. When the blanket was out you might need to think a bit, but eventually you could figure out there was a flaw in his routine.

Floyd was always provided a treat sometime before we went to bed. One night I forgot to provide this treat. The next morning, I arose to the blanket located near where his treat bag was stored. When he was really concerned about a situation, he would drag his entire bed out for inspection. Once when I purchased a different treat for him, he dragged the whole bed out. It took awhile, but we figured it out.

There was always a good reason for his behavior.

He would sometimes look at you in manner that let you know he was either not feeling well, or he was not happy with you. This occurred when I had him neutered. Hours after the neutering, he obviously was not feeling well. However, after he was more aware of his surroundings, he spent a few days looking at me like, "What was the purpose in doing this?" He looked at me out of the corner of his eye and avoided me. After these few days, he finally interacted with me again.

The first week in October each year, I went bow hunting for deer in the lower Upper Peninsula of Michigan with my friends, who owned a cabin there. The first two years Floyd lived with us, he decided to protest my leaving for this trip by pooping in areas he delegated for this purpose. He would not do this on the carpet but would find places where his untidy "leavings" were not difficult to clean up.

He would wait for me to come home from work at the front door at the time I usually came home. When this did not happen, he would later perform the dirty deed. At no other time did he do these odd jobs around the house. When I returned home, I would get the "look" for a few days. After this two-year period, Floyd still waited at the door, but the so-called protest did not follow. He seemed to realize also that I would be home eventually, so the sulking when I returned never developed again. When I left for conferences for work, he also understood that I was going to return.

Floyd shared our life for twelve years. He never stopped waiting at our door when the time came to come home from work. If I was late, he would walk the floor until my return. Once I returned, he greeted me with his standard wag of the tail.

Floyd, as I said, was a very cordial fellow. On one occasion, a friend of ours knocked on our door. My wife was in the back portion of our house and did not hear our friend enter the front room and be greeted by Floyd. Our friend asked Floyd if he knew where my wife was. Floyd ushered her back to where my wife was using her sewing machine. He very much knew good people and those to mistrust.

On a wintry Sunday, we came home from church, and Floyd would not settle down. He kept running around. We had left the door unlocked. My wife said, "He is trying to tell us something." About a half-hour later, a sheriff deputy arrived to tell us someone had been seen leaving our house while we were gone. Come to find out, it was a youth that had escaped from a youth retention home and was on the run with his girlfriend, and they had entered our house to get warm.

The only thing that ever set Floyd off was when he saw birds. He barked at them. If you heard him bark, nine chances out of ten, a bird was nearby. He would look out the window sometimes and run around barking after he spied one. For the most part though, Floyd lived as Snoopy said, "No sense in doing a lot of barking if you don't really have anything to say."

Floyd always felt pooping was a private matter. When you let him out to do his deed, he preferred that you did not watch him. He'd find a spot that was secluded if you accompanied him. I would let him out in the winter, and he would not venture too far from our house. He would be slow to have a movement if you stood watching him. He would look at you like, "Do you need to watch me do this?" Therefore, we tried to leave him alone during these events.

My youngest daughter would come visit us with her dog, a schnauzer, named Bonzie. Bonzie was allowed on the furniture. Every time he showed up, Floyd would look at us like, "What's the deal here!" He never took any action to protest. He just flowed with the moment and played with Bonzie. Bonzie was born on September 11, 2001, in Virginia Beach, Virginia. He was born on a day with history. Bonzie was also a very good dog, so he and Floyd played well together.

Floyd loved to go to the groomer every other month. When he came home from his first sessions, the groomer would put a kerchief of different colors around his neck. I told him he looked like a sissy with these cloth units on. After a few times, he seemed to get what I was saying. My wife thought he looked cute with them on. After my wife picked him up from the groomer, he would run around the house with his kerchief on. When I arrived home, he walked sheepishly toward me with his head bowed. I would take the kerchief off, and he would bounce around again. Therefore he pleased us both.

We purchased one-half of the cabin in northern Michigan in 2003. I had accompanied my friends to the cabin for several years. Floyd went with us to the cabin each time we visited for 2004-2008. We always had a good time with him at the cabin, because we could spend quality time with him.

Floyd only had one reprieve from the furniture. He could sit in my chair beside me for as long as he wanted to each day. He would jump up beside me for a short period of time, depending on his needs. He would sit there proud as a peacock and look at my wife in a manner that indicated he felt he was getting away with something.

In 2006, he developed arthritis in his back legs. This progressed to the point where he had more and more trouble getting around. I needed to help him get up in my chair.

One morning in April of 2006, he could hardly walk. I took him to the vet and she gave me medicine to give him and told me to build a ramp for him to be placed where the steps existed. This was my first realization that Floyd's life was limited to just a few more years. I decided to put it out of my mind, not wanting to think about it. He got better after this, but he would not walk on the ramp. He would position himself so he could make it up the steps on his own. He was a determined little guy, not giving in to his handicap.

On Christmas Day 2007, as our family was sitting around talking, my son-in-law and I commented how matter was projecting from Floyd's eyes. My wife said, "Oh, he gets that once in a while." He seemed lethargic also. We needed to renew his license in January 2008. I said jokingly that maybe Floyd would not live another three years, which was the term of the license.

Floyd continued to slow down. I thought it was as a result of growing older. I could not foresee the news we received the first week in March 2008. My wife took him to the vet for his routine checkup. He required shots and the vet did an additional test.

When I returned home from work that day, my wife said, "I have some terrible news. Floyd has cancer and has about three weeks to live." I began to cry. I was shocked at the news. We were told to give him some medicine, which would comfort him. The vet said we would know when it was time, and probably we would need to put him down when the time came. She said he probably would lose his ability to hold water and his stool.

My wife visited the vet on a Monday. Floyd weakened a bit thereafter, but he still followed his daily routine. At first I thought the vet might be wrong. The second Friday after the checkup he started to show signs of going downhill fast. Saturday, he continued to get worse. When we left for church Sunday morning, he seemed to be better; he even had a spring in his step. When we returned home, he was going downhill even more. His breathing became stressed. At 4:00 p.m. I called the vet, who was on call. He said it sounded like it would not be long now and to bring him in to our regular doctor on Monday morning for final action.

We hugged Floyd several times and talked to him as much as possible. Floyd never messed in the house during this period. He continued to do his duty outside. A short time after 8:00 p.m., he indicated he wanted to go outside. I followed him along the way. He went under a pine tree we have in our front yard. He peed, he hesitated, and then went down to his knees. I picked him up and carried him back in the house. Just as we passed through the kitchen, he stiffened his body licked me, and then proceeded to pass away.

Floyd never licked anyone; he was not a kissing type of dog. He showed his love in so many other ways. Just the sparkle in his eyes and how he made you feel was oh, so great. If you had a bad day, Floyd was always there to cheer you up.

When I came home from work the next day we buried him in our back yard with the MSU blanket and some of his favorite toys. My wife purchased a round, flat cement decorative stone, and we placed it on his grave. We received several notes of sympathy from people who knew Floyd and those who knew how much we loved him.

I have a theory. When you find a pet like Floyd who you discover you have a special bond with, love grows within you and the pet. As the bonding grows each day and week into years, the pet becomes one with you. I did not believe some of the stories I have heard from pet owners about their pets until Floyd came along. He was my dog, my buddy, and my pal. He also communicated well with my wife. My wife was just as upset when he died as I was

When Floyd died, I watched the human spirit factor leave him. His body became, hence, a common animal cadaver. This, however, is just my theory. This is an example that when the book of life is written, the answers are not in the back of the book.

Joey and Fido were excellent pets, but Floyd was so extra special.

Red Foley, a country singer of my childhood and prior years, was the author of the following song that says a lot about special dogs:

# Old Shep

When I was a lad
And old Shep was a pup
Over hills and meadows we'd stray
Just a boy and his dog
We were both full of fun
We grew up together that way

I remember a time at the old swimmin' hole
When I would have drowned beyond doubt
But old Shep was right there.
To the rescue he came
He jumped in and then pulled me out

As the years fast did roll
Old Shep, he grew old
His eyes were fast growing dim
And one day the doctor looked at me and said
"I can't do no more for him, Jim"

With a hand that was trembling
I picked up my gun
And aimed it at Shep's faithful head
I just couldn't do it, I wanted to run
I wish they would shoot me instead

He came to my side and looked up at me
And laid his old head on my knee
I had struck the best friend a man ever had
I cried so I scarcely could see

Oh Shep, he has gone where the good doggies go
And no more with old Shep will I roam
But if dogs have a heaven there's one thing I know
Old Shep has a wonderful home

# TALE NINETEEN

## The Comedians

A S I MENTIONED IN MY introduction, my uncle Will and my cousin Norm inspired me to always try to have a story available for sharing in a humorous manner. Uncle Will was my father's brother, and cousin Norm was related to me on my mother's side.

My uncle Will was a very meticulous farmer. He had a very well-kept farm with impeccable livestock and machinery. His house, barn, and outbuildings were picturesque. His wife, my aunt of course, was a saintly woman. I do not remember ever hearing her say an injurious word about anyone. In fact, if someone said something not so complimentary about someone she would comment, "Forevermore, I did not know that about them," or 'Forevermore, I never encountered that in my dealings with him or her." This would not insult the person who made the comment or the person being discussed. In most cases, the person would lessen the demeaning remarks. She died of lung cancer in the mid 1960s although she had never smoked a day in her life. It took my uncle almost two years to get back to his old self. There was no storytelling during this period. Slowly, after this period, he started enjoying life again and began telling his stories again.

My cousin Norm could repair anything. He operated an auto repair business, sold televisions, repaired televisions, and helped my uncle the DeKalb salesman farm 120 acres of land.

Both my uncle and cousin would tell stories about experiences they had in their life and would throw in a joke that may fit within the story. Many of the stories were geared toward the person's personality, and you would need to know them. If you did not fully know the person, they would preface the story with a description of the individual. The stories were never hurtful.

The manner in which they presented the story provided a high percentage of the enjoyment you could have listening to the tales. I could not do them justice relating the stories, so I will only relate some of the jokes they told. I do not know the source of these jokes but I have heard some of them again, since they told them a number of times. Some I have never heard again.

Most farmers did not show much love for a milk inspector. In fact, when I described to some of my relatives, who were farmers, what I did for a living after I completed my college education (I became a health department official), they questioned my sanity, but they also accepted it- though one relative said with enjoyment in his voice that my dad would roll over in his grave if he knew what I was doing.

Uncle Will told a joke a number of times about a milk inspector who visited a farm. The milk inspector showed the farmer his card which identified him. He told the farmer, "That card allows me to inspect any portion of this farm and your operations that I wish to observe." The inspector proceeded to inspect a salt block. (It is commonplace in many barnyards for cows to lick salt as part of their diet.) A bull came on the scene and began chasing the inspector around the barnyard. As the inspector passed the farmer, who was standing outside the fence boarding the area, for the third time, the inspector asked the farmer, "What should I do?" The farmer said, "Show him your card."

The city twelve miles southeast of our farm had many Irish Catholics residing there. A rivalry existed between the Irish from this group and the Germans of Southwest Town. Each sect would tell jokes about the other. My uncle Will told a joke about an Irishman and a German who applied for the same job. The owner of the business was an Irishman. They were given a test with twenty questions. Both scored nineteen out of twenty. The German was given the job. The Irish applicant asked the owner why the German was picked over him, since they scored the same on the test and he shared the same nationality as the owner. The owner said, "Because on question six the German answered, "I do not know," and you answered "I do not know either." (When my dad died, my mother, sister, and I became members of the Irish parish. As the years went by, many Germans and Irish married. A rivalry in sports still remains to this day.)

Cousin Norm:

There was a preacher in a town. The preacher was told there was a farmer who might not be saved. He lived three miles out of town. The preacher went out to speak with the man, or at least have a discussion with him, about the Lord. The preacher came upon the farmer out in his field. The preacher said to the farmer, "Oh, I see you are working on the fruits of the Lord's vineyard."

The farmer said, "These are soybeans, not grapes."

The preacher said, "I know; it's from the Bible. Are you a Christian?"

The farmer said, "My name is Homer Smith. You're looking for Jim Christian; he lives two miles south of here."

The preacher said, "No, are you lost?"

The farmer said, "No, I have lived here all my life."

The preacher said, "Do you know about the day of resurrection?"

The farmer said, "When is it going to be?"

The preacher said, "Today, tomorrow, or the next day."

The farmer said, "Don't tell my wife; she will want to go all three days."

Cousin Norm:

A couple were married twenty-five years. The wife said, "Why don't we butcher a pig and celebrate with our friends and relatives."

The husband said, "Why should a pig sacrifice his life for a mistake we made twenty-five years ago!"

Uncle Will:

A man drove in a ditch accidently in front of a farmer's home. The farmer retrieved his horse and led him to the site. The farmer said to the horse, "Pull, Jack, pull." The horse did not move. The farmer said to the horse, "Pull, Dolly, pull!" The horse did not move. The famer said to the horse, "Pull, Buck, pull!" The horse did not move. The farmer said to the horse, "Pull, Buddy, pull." The horse pulled the car out.

The man asked why he called the horse the wrong names first before calling him by the right one. The farmer said, "Buddy is blind, so if he thought he was the only one pulling, he would never pull."

Cousin Norm:

A man's car broke down near a farm. He was looking under the hood of the car when a cow left the other cows in the pasture and came near the fence that contained them. The cow said to the man that he probably had a plugged fuel pump and that a service station was within three miles of the farm.

The man, astonished that a cow could talk, rushed up to the farmhouse and knocked on the door. The man explained that the cow had talked to him. The farmer said, "Was she brown with white spots?" The man said, "Yes, she was."

The farmer said, "She does not know anything about cars. The black one with the white spots around the head, now that cow knows cars. I would rely on what she says."

Uncle Will:

A couple were married six months when the woman's mother came to visit their farm. The woman could not find anything right about what the farmer was doing with the farm. When they were going through the barn, the woman got too close to the farmer's bull and was kicked in the head, and she passed on.

At the funeral, the preacher witnessed that when women came up to the man, he would hug them and nod his head in the affirmative. When the men came up, he would shake his head negatively and shake hands with them. Finally the preacher approached the man and asked him what was going on when the women and the men approached him.

The man said when the women approached him, they would say how terrible it was how she died. He said he hugged them and told them yes, it was. When the men approached, they would ask if they could borrow the bull. He told them no, he was booked up for a year.

Cousin Norm:

A farmer was standing out in his wheat field each night until it got dark. A man who witnessed this every day stopped one day to ask him what he was doing. The farmer said he wanted to win the Nobel Prize. The man said, "What does standing in your wheat field have to do with winning the Nobel Prize?" The farmer said, "They say in order to win the Nobel Prize, you must be outstanding in your field."

Uncle Will:

There was a farmer around our area that always bragged about how much land he owned. The farmer commented for some time that it took at least a half-hour to drive his truck around all parts of his land. One Sunday after church, he was going on again. My uncle Will said, "I had a truck like that once too, but I got rid of it."

Cousin Norm:

Norm told a story about a guy who made a fur coat for his wife out of two German shepherd dog skins. The dogs had been killing chickens. He said every night that she went out for a special affair with the coat on, she was putting on the dog.

# Tale Twenty

# One Altar Service

AT THE BEGINNING OF MARCH in my fifth year of school, all the boys in our class were detained from recess to discuss becoming an assistant to the priest at Catholic Mass. A nun who was in charge of the program informed us we would need to learn Latin prayers and phrases to qualify to become an altar server. She said a series of sessions would be held with her to go over the proper actions to perform during the Mass, and we would spend time with the priest going over the vestments which were worn for a Mass and other ceremonies, plus the instruments that would be used.

At first my interest was not piqued in performing this activity. My mother and father were excited about the thought of my character building if I became a server. The thought patterns of a fifth grader could change from day to day. I knew I could pass muster in learning the vestments and implements required during Mass, but learning the Latin prayers and phrases alarmed me. Playground activities and home play were number one on my interest chart.

Once per week you could make an appointment with the program manager, Sister Mary Blank. She would affirm whether you qualified as a server. When the first four boys made the grade and I observed them serving their first Mass, I became more interested. One of the boys was my second cousin who was a first cousin to the Pioneer Corn salesman's son. The second was the fellow who had been pushed down the steps entering the cafeteria. These two had a history of being first in everything. They were very capable students and had our teachers wrapped around their fingers. They were above average in ability to learn. They, however, would take advantage of their reputation and would take shortcuts depending on the task.

Example: We received pins for the number of books we read during the year in our fourth year of school. There were levels at which you could receive larger more valued pins, depending on the number of books you read. If you read one hundred books, you would receive a plaque.

These two characters would write book reports by scanning the book and reading the jacket information regarding the book. They received credit for reading close to 125 books that year and were awarded a special honor at the end of the year. I read about forty books, as I remember, but I read them cover to cover and enjoyed their contents.

They bragged about their methods to some of us, but, being honorable, we did not blow the whistle on them. Since they excelled in so many other things, it probably would not have done any good to tattle on them. They always received the benefit of the doubt.

After seeing the first four boys perform their duties as altar boys, I wanted to be a server. Therefore I began studying. I worked hard. I asked my sister and mother to run through the prayers and phrases with me. I seemed to do well when I recited them with them. But when I went over them with the project manager, I failed to meet her standards. She would not give me any leeway. My history of being a roustabout did not aid me. The nun in charge as much as told me that my citizenship did not classify me for the honor of being a server.

The second week in May was the last week to qualify. After failing to qualify the first week in May, the evaluator told me maybe I should wait until the following year. I was determined to make the grade. I studied even harder. The second week in May, I made the grade.

I was placed with the two smart boys and another first-time qualifier to serve for a week before school ceremonies. My folks were very proud of me and attended my first Mass service.

There was a long prayer at the beginning of Mass which was called the Creed. The first words were recited by the priest and continued by the server. I noticed that although, I was saying the prayer clearly, the two "angels" were mumbling this prayer and a few other phrases throughout the Mass.

After Mass, our priest asked the two "top dogs" and me to meet with him. The priest said, "I told you two boys the last time you served to learn your prayers better." He further said, "You should learn your prayers as well as this young gentleman." The second and third day they did not do much better. Our priest made them stop and start over at the beginning prayer three or four times. Their response was not much better to a few other prayers.

After the third Mass, our priest said, "Tell Sister Blank to have two other boys serve the remaining two services, and you will not serve again until you can recite the prayers correctly." They eventually got their act together, and I served with them several times after that.

I served at many Catholic functions and events, including weddings and funerals at both the Irish and German parishes. I also served at functions at other churches for my relatives.

Three serving events, however, stand out in my memory. The first occurred the summer between seventh and eighth grade at my school training life at Southwestern school. Three boys and I were scheduled to serve a week of ceremonies. A visiting priest came to our parish to conduct Mass for the week. In those days, Catholics were not allowed to share in the wine. The priest actually used the water and wine twice during the ceremony. The priest usually brought a limited amount of water and wine in two separate cruets.

The visiting priest brought two large cruets. One was filled halfway with water, and the other was filled to the brim with wine. He would bring the cruets into our dressing area where the cassocks were kept. The priest would use the entire contents of the wine cruet. We could not believe the amount of wine he would garner from the cruet.

On the fourth day, we decided to take a small sip of the wine. We added a bit of the water to replace what we took. The test of the wine wasn't worth our while. The excitement of doing something out of the ordinary was more fulfilling. At our age, we could not understand how this visiting priest could drink so much of that bitter substance.

The second event was the first time I served a Mass for a funeral. This event occurred during my eighth year of elementary school. The funeral was for an older man who did not have any young relatives. The three boys and I were summoned to serve. Not one of us had served at a funeral before. Our priest was a stickler for exact procedures. He made no bones about dressing you down in front of everyone, so we were nervous to begin with.

At the beginning of the service, the priest went around the casket with a censer, blessing the body with incense. One of my co-servers, who was to follow the priest around as part of the ritual, managed to trip him. All of us managed to follow in his footsteps, so to speak, making additional mistakes at one time or other.

I was required to circle the church with a crucifix mounted on a metal rod for all to observe. I was not watching carefully when I approached the archway in the back of the church and knocked the crucifix off its pedestal by striking the top of the archway. This caused one or two people in attendance to laugh. After this we began snickering out of embarrassment for our actions. After the ceremony in church, we rode to the cemetery in our priest's car for final burial prayers and procedures. He did not say a word on the way.

One of my comrades dropped the wand used for blessing the body on the ground during the procedures at this location. The mistake again caused snickering among the chosen four. When we returned from the cemetery, our priest told us to tell Sister Blank to never send any one of us to serve a funeral again. He said, "You were a disgrace to your parents, your school, and our parish."

The third episode happened on a Sunday, the summer of 1960. We always had a ceremony called Benediction after the 10:30 a.m. Mass. Catholics know that this ceremony consists of singing a hymn at the beginning, saying a litany of prayers, singing another hymn, performing a blessing with proper instruments, and singing another hymn at the end.

A short time prior to the ending of Mass, a server would place a small, scented, charcoal briquette in a censer with a little incense. This mixture would be lit and allowed to burn. Our priest, for some reason, always wanted to create an abundance of fumes throughout the church. We servers always tried our best to accommodate him, but he always seem to discredit our attempts.

I was the designated one this day to light the censer. I placed an overabundant amount of incense in the bowl of the censer. The charcoal was red hot when I brought it out to conduct the proceedings. The method we were taught, to properly direct the censer, was to always create a large arc when swinging the unit back and forth. The outcome of the swinging was to create a flurry of incense. The swinging of the unit was a continuous process only to be interrupted by a short blessing with the sacred tool. After the priest added incense to the bowl, they sang the second hymn.

I decided this day, since the censor was burning excellently, to increase the arc of the swing. The execution of this process created an excitement of the mixture that spread to the front four or five pews of the church. A sheet of fog separated the parishioners behind these seats. I thought surely when it came time for the priest to take the action of adding the additional incense, he would not add any or very little. He added the normal portion. When I went back to my post to swing the censer, I continued my efforts to see how large an arc I could master and how much haze I could create.

By the end of the service, I had created a cloud of incense to the back of the church.

Our priest did not complain after the ceremony on this occasion about the lack of fumes I generated, nor did he comment regarding any overabundance. When I got in our car to travel home, Dad asked me, "What were you doing with all the incense in church? Didn't Father get upset with you?" I told him that he never mentioned a word about it. My dad said, "Don't try that again."

The next day at school, all my friends who had attended the Mass commended me for the feat. I took my dad's advice, however, and in the future no one ever tried to match or better my performance.

# TALE TWENTY-ONE

## Two Chores

I N THE DAYS OF MY youth every farm boy, when he turned six to eight years old, depending on the number of his older brothers, was drafted into helping with chores. Every day of the week throughout the entire year, the chores needed to be done. Feeding and watering chickens, gathering eggs, milking, and bedding cows were daily chores. In addition, there was cleaning cow barns and chicken coops by removing manure before placing bedding down. Cleaning milking implements, feeding and bedding horses, feeding pigs, and cleaning pigpens were chores. Gathering eggs occurred once per day; milking cows occurred twice per day. When calves were born, they needed special treatment.

When I was between six and eight, I mostly took care of calf maintenance and gathering the eggs. This was "helping" with chores. Feeding and bedding after my father performed some preliminary gathering of these items to the area of the feeding bins and bedding areas for animals was being helpful with chores.

Weaning a calf from the mother could be a interesting experience. When a calf would first drink out of a pail, for a while their entire head would be submerged in the pail with the calf's nose touching the bottom of the pail. The calf would then ease off to lap the milk. The calf would butt the pail, following its prior methods of retrieving the milk as it did from the mother's udder. Holding the pail steady so milk did not spill was an effort for a young man of six to eight years of age. Sometimes the bovine offspring's head would become airborne when butting against the side of the pail and fly recklessly. You would need to watch carefully that your privates remained untouched.

My father discussed this issue with me. My first painful experience in this regard that I can remember was when I was about four years old. It involved the pump handle on the hand pump. I was circumcised when

115

I was a few days old, so I do not remember that experience, but my first experience regarding getting slammed in the crotch area will always stand out. A partner jumping off of a seesaw when he or she had me elevated in the air also was a defining moment in the world of being smacked in this area.

Knowing this, I let my guard down one day, however, and I was standing bracing myself against the pail as a calf was drinking from the pail. Suddenly the calf came up and nailed me. Ouch! Ouch! The pail went one way, the calf went another way, and I went to my knees. My dad asked me what was wrong, as he had not been close by when the painful event occurred. Since I had been warned, I did not wish to supply any pertinent information regarding what had transpired, so I slowly remarked the standard, "Oh nothing, the calf wanted to play or something." He said, "Oh... well, be careful."

After the pain subsided, I managed to walk bowlegged to where my dad was milking a cow. He provided an adequate amount of milk to feed the calf. I think he knew my concern but did not let on. I gathered the calf and continued assisting in its feeding. In the future, I learned to stay seated on a stool instead of standing when feeding a calf. This method protected my privates, and, learning the proper leverage, I could still be in control of the situation. It also helped in learning to hold your ground in a sporting contest.

When I explained my plight to my friends in school regarding this incident, although they had gone through the same ordeal themselves, they still found it to be hilarious. It is rather interesting that we all find the discussion of this temporary distress and any encounter with anything to do with hemorrhoids to be a source of humor. As long as you are not the victim, those stories are a fountain of laughter.

A friend of mine was kicked in the groin area in football on one occasion in high school. When he gained some ability to walk off the field, the last thing he wanted to do was to comfort his injury with his hands. So he walked off the field bent over with his hands on his thighs. The announcer said, "I believe he must have a back or upper leg injury." His fellow teammates found the incident to be a source of humor then and for future discussions.

On one occasion when I was playing third base for our high school team, an opponent hit a line drive. It managed to seek out my crotch area. I successfully made the throw for a force-out of the runner going to second base. Thank the Lord, it was the last out of the inning, so I had some time to gather myself, so to speak. As usual, the laughter was uniform among my teammates.

Our baseball diamond was about a half mile from our school through our downtown area. After the game was over, trying to be brave, I decided not to take my coach's offer to have someone transport me to the school by car. The walk was a journey to remember. A number of people were curious to know why I was walking in the manner I was. My answer was to chide, "Oh, I pulled a muscle in my thigh." This, of course, brought on more humorous comments from my teammates who accompanied me. The results of the occasion, however, left me with a black-and-blue color in the relevant area for about a week. My gait was also slowed a bit.

Every man or boy has had similar experiences as I have documented here.

Like most farm boys, I had a fondness for animals. Each cow we owned had a name in those days. Chickens were too numerous to name, much like today's herds of cattle who are housed in large facilities for mass production of milk. For that matter, it was not good to get too close to roosters, since they serve no purpose but to be the first butchered from a new flock of chickens, for Sunday dinner or special occasions.

I was not summoned to the barn or chicken coop in the morning until I reached the age of ten, as only milking occurred at this time. Before the age of ten, I had not yet achieved the level of maturity to approach a cow's udders with safety. The only time I was allowed to do so was under close supervision.

The egg gathering was not performed by me, of course, when I was attending school; my mother performed these duties in my absence. Weekends and vacations from school were my times to perform this duty.

Advancement to handling manure and pitching hay were added to my chores when I reached the golden age of ten. About this time, my fondness for the creatures I tended to was curtailed, but for the most part I still liked animals and being around them.

The turning of a furrow with a plow for planting of crops, the smell of freshly mixed soil after disking and using another implement to "drag" a field, watching seeds grow into plants, watching eggs being laid, and filling a pail with milk from a cow-these gifts of farming helped bridle any anguish with days of chores.

My dad did not enjoy the television much apart from watching Lawrence Welk. He enjoyed music as much as anything, so he always had a radio in the barn playing music while we did chores. He would sometimes sing along with the songs. He had a wonderful voice but was very reticent about when and where he sang. He would sing in church or once in a while when Mom played the piano, and in the barn. The "herd" of cows seemed to enjoy it when they "heard" him sing here and there throughout the barn. The music would eliminate the boredom of listening to cows munch on alfalfa and the mooing from the cows, softening the snorting of horses, the rattling of stanchions, and the blowing of the cold winter wind outside the barn.

Milking a cow builds up muscles in the forearms. Pitching hay out a haymow with loose or baled hay, pitching it down a hay chute and then placing it the manger of each cow works on a variety of muscles.

My dad milked cows by hand, so milking machines were not available. The back and knees were not tested very much with milking machines. Sitting on a stool manipulating the cows' teats was more of strain to the back and the knees for my father than for me, since I was more agile at my age.

The sound of the milk hitting the pail, listening to easy-listening music, and leaning against the cow mesmerizes you. However, the calm mood could quickly be bitterly broken by a dry or gutter-soaked tail swatted sharply to the head or face. We had one cow who had a penchant for creating this occupational hazard. My dad had a string contraption he attached to her tail and then on her legs that eliminated this menace. The other cows were more devious. You never knew when a random tail would fly in your direction. A slap in the face caused duels in bygone days, so it was human nature to be most furious, prompting a backlash of various forms of vocal rage. My dad did not tolerate swearing, but a hard slap with hand on the cow's leg or butt with a Jack Benny-like comment, "Now cut that out! " in a stern voice was promoted. When similar circumstances presented themselves in other barns in the surrounding area, the gestures and language were probably much more crude. Most people would be so upset after they were hit that they would probably tie the tail down, meaning they were "fit to be tied."

I usually milked one or two cows during the evening session up until the *Flintstones* hit the airwaves. On the night the *Flintstones* were on, I was beckoned to milk a few more cows. I would quicken my step a bit more regarding other chores and take on more assignments so my dad would not miss this program.

The Rosary was recited together as a family after supper during Advent and Lent. Supper was served earlier on the *Flintstones* night during this time. My sister or I always led the prayers of the Rosary. If one of us tried to travel too quickly in our leadership, Dad would stop us and say, "Slow down and think about the words you are reciting." On the *Flintstone* nights, a little haste set the pace; he made no comments if we hurried as long as we did not get out of hand. Unfortunately, Dad passed away after a couple seasons of the *Flintstones* had been completed.

My dad raised pigs for slaughter for our own use during my younger years, but discontinued the development of pork in about 1955. My parents decided that purchasing pork over the meat counter occasionally was cheaper than raising them. I did get in on the tail end of feeding the swine wormy apples, weeds, and waste from food products. I never had to clean the pens of these wallowing and ill-mannered, mud-loving beasts. Chicken manure ran a close second to pig manure, which won the first-place trophy for odor when cleaning after the occupants.

Watching the methods of butchering pigs and cows in those days was repelling. The methods today, I feel, are more humane, although some might disagree. Our method of ending a chicken's life gave me firsthand observation to the term "running around like a chicken with its head cut off."

I did find the steps taken from bringing the animal to slaughter to processing the carcass for the purpose of consuming the meat to be very educational. The comparisons years later regarding better standards in processing were also intriguing. In my thirty-six years of work for health agencies, I witnessed several breakthroughs in more beneficial methods of raising, processing, storing, and holding meat products. Discovering that feeding raw garbage to pigs was not appropriate, since it increased the chances of illness, was one. Some of the changes in the methods have also created the need for a closer watchful eye, such as mass processing of meats, where animals never see the light of day.

My father's first job when he was sixteen years of age was working for a farmer who raised sheep. My dad and others found sheep to be lovable but dimwitted. My dad never discredited any animal except a sheep. He said they were the dumbest animals on the face of the earth. He said they could walk off and not find their way back. Then when you went to guide them, they fought you every step of the way, attempting to wander off more. The use of sheepdogs was no advantage he said. "They were more trouble than they were worth," he said.

One Sunday when I was twelve, my semi-genius second cousin and the Pioneer salesman's son came over to my house together with the semi-genius's dad. We hit a few baseballs to each other and progressed to walking back to our woods to check out any wildlife.

When we returned from the woods, one of us, I can't remember which one, suggested we attempt to ride three five-to-six-week old calves. The calves were more than happy to oblige us; bucking, kicking, and squirming to get us off their backs. Although the dismissals from their backs incurred a number of shots to our bodies, any discussion of chickening out was not an option.

Just as I was being tossed off a young heifer's back, my father entered the barn to witness my final landing onto a cow pie. This ended our idea of fun. A lecture was forthcoming regarding the health of both the calves and ourselves by performing such shenanigans. My cousins left very quickly thereafter. We were all left with minor bumps and bruises, which we did not dare discuss with our parents.

Each year since I could remember we ordered three hundred Leghorn chicks, which arrived by mail in boxes of fifty chicks to a box. A second delivery from the post office was instituted for those days when farmers ordered these birds in the spring of the year.

We placed them in a small housing unit called a brooder house. This unit contained a heating device centered with a oval-brimmed metal hood that extended about eighteen inches in all directions from the heater. The heater was fueled with kerosene. The biddies huddled around the heater instinctively when we placed them in the brooder house. We always lost a few chicks each year for one reason or another. The brooder house had to be built airtight to guard against the entrance of wildlife predators looking for an easy meal.

I really enjoyed watching the chicks grow into pullets and young roosters. It was amazing to behold the short time it took for these little biddies to mature into a fully grown bird.

Six to eight weeks after their arrival on the scene a less-than-fun task awaited us. The chickens' wings needed to be clipped to reduce the height that they could achieve when they attempted to fly. This was performed by my dad in the brooder house, and then the birds would be transported to the chicken coop by my sister, my mother, and I. Once they were clipped, they were gathered and carried by their legs. Normally we carried two birds in each hand on the journey from the brooder house to the chicken coop. They would flap their wings as you carried them. This necessitated the wearing of gloves and long-sleeved clothing; otherwise, the freshly clipped wings would cut the skin. Even with the protective clothing, once in awhile a sharpened wing would sneak between an opening between a glove and sleeve. The last year before my father died I did some clipping of wings; the flapping of wings was just as active when this task was performed. When this task was completed, a sigh of relief was given by all participants, including the chickens.

It was fun to go into our chicken coop just after dark; the chickens would roost in the upper area perch-type units that lined the north portion of our coop. The chickens would sing in a humming style. It was a very soothing sound.

# A Break in the Prose
# At a Loss for Who Won

Our opponents were they and they prevailed
Their opponents were them and they prevailed
They opposed eight teams of them and they prevailed
Their opponents in the final contest were another team of them
They were conquered by them

We defeated the team of them who defeated they on two
occasions during the defined season

The victorious team of them were considered the finest of the
land
They were regarded and typecast as losers

They participated three years in a row in the final event
The team of them had not reached the final event ever in the
history of the final event

Who was the loser?
Are they really losers?
Are we losers?
Are we winners because we think of them as winners even though
we soundly defeated them?

Maybe those who watched us, they and them, are the overall
winners
Maybe us, they, and them being able to compete for the prize
should be considered winners

Struggling, striving, experiencing heartbreak along the way might
be the reward

Win or lose, the effort might be longer-lasting when looking back
at the achievement.

# Mastering a Reaction

Off the coast of Portland, Maine
A Man, a tall Man
A Woman, a small Woman
A Dog, a curious Dog
A Seagull, a soaring Seagull
A Boat, an Incoming Sailboat
All met at the same point
On a rainy day

The water was rough and chopping
Just the day before, still water had a strong undertow
The Man, the Dog, the Seagull, and the boats firsthand
Were no strangers to the wind and rain
The Woman, when sheltered, loved the sound of rain

The Dog smelled the air
With the lift of his nose

The Seagull made a unsteady landing

The Boat fast approaching
Realized nature's abrupt showing of its power
Of who was in charge

The Man scooped up the Woman
To take her to safer
Means of viewing

Nature forever will be a mystery

A Dog was made to withstand some of nature's uproars
Learning to seek shelter when the need be
Taming by man has left it more vulnerable

The Seagull knows all manners to contend with
Nature's moments of trial and loving touch
The Seagull can be hurt most by man's disregard for
Nature's treasures with pollution

A Sailboat can make use of nature's winds for its
Forward move to get from here to there or to compete for
enjoyment
But nature's commotion can render it helpless
When winds become out of control

The human with its reasoning power
Should be the least in danger
However, the human mind plays tricks
Therefore to some humans fighting nature is a challenge
When safety may be the best solution
No matter, the stature and bravery rings more true

# Love Hurts

You can forget there are two ways that love falls
We have the right to error once in awhile
Out of love and in love
A sharing must take place by two

One in and one out
Hurts both if when two were there once
The one in can be fooled at first
Thinking mutual love will return
Laughing it off will turn into sadness
Time may or may not be the cure

The first time many times hurts most
It can last a lifetime in some cases
Friendship covers scars
After the wounds heal

Lifetime absences can leave open wounds
Wounds that an occasional chat or chance meeting would heal
Healing of a precious memory that lingers.

# TALE TWENTY-TWO

## Transportation

I AM NOT SURE WHEN THE horse-and-buggy days ended for my mother and dad. My mom's family, I know, used a semi-covered wagon that my grandfather constructed for their journey in 1914, when they moved to the area where my mom grew up. The move was made when my mom was one year old.

My dad's father died when my dad was fifteen years old, in 1919. I never heard whether my dad's father ever owned a car. My dad started working on the sheep farm at sixteen, but I do not know when he began riding in or driving a motorized vehicle.

Model T Fords were around in those days (known as Tin Lizzies). Model A's came into existence in 1927. My mother told a story about a driving experience her dad had. I do not know the year of the encounter; I know the car he drove was a Model A, so the experience must have been after 1927.

My grandfather, I guess, had just purchased the vehicle; I do not know whether it was new. He decided to head into town to visit my grandmother's brother. Now my grandmother's brother and my grandfather were really close. They made beer together from a German recipe. My mother related that when these two would tap the container they held the beer in while brewing and storing, some of the barrel's contents were so unfit…they would shoot above the windmill that towered over all the buildings on their property. I presume from hearing some of their motivations that no one knew what they may indulge in next.

After spending a short period of time together discussing issues, one issue evidently caused a difference of opinion. The source of their argument never was established. My grandfather left his brother-in-law's house in a huff.

After Grandfather was home for a short time, he had some remorse. He decided to head back into town to apologize to my mother's uncle. By this time it was getting dark enough to have your car lamps lit. My mother's uncle evidently experienced the same feelings, so he opted to head out to my grandfather's farm. According to my mother, neither man ever motored faster than ten to fifteen miles per hour. At some point between the two destinations, they managed to run into each other. Apparently my grandfather thought he had his light attachment engaged, but it was not out far enough. The newness of the car probably was the reasoning for his error.

When the small cloud of dust settled, my mother's uncle yelled in German from his car, "Where are your lights!" When my grandpa got out of his car, he must have bumped the device just enough to allow the lights to blink. Therefore my grandpa said in German, "Lights, I got lights, lights, I got lights." This caused a short debate with words from both that had little clarity to those who gathered. Legend has it that Grandpa did not have his lights on at the time my two relatives came together, but my grandpa was not convinced. The damage was very minimal, so I heard.

I understand, after a couple of days to cool off, the two men began talking to each other again and collaborated on repairing their cars. Mom said it was just an excuse to have a beer, as the damage to either vehicle was hardly visible.

I do know that the vehicle that my dad had when my parents were first married was a 1931 Model A Ford (the last year they were made). I have no idea when he purchased the car. I also know that Democrats in our area during this time purchased Fords and Republicans purchased Chevrolets. The people in the township we lived in, and immediate surrounding area, were almost all Democrats. The township supervisor, my uncle, was a Democrat, and all other officials were Democrats, except my cousin the Pioneer corn salesman, who was a Republican. He was the township clerk. My uncle the postmaster drove a Chevrolet. He was a Republican.

In 1946 just before I entered this world, my dad bought a 1942 Ford coupe. This car had two regular seats in the front portion and two small, padded seats which were attached to the inner sides of the car behind the front seats. There was a flat area between the seats where a small child could sit and lean back against the stuffed attachment that came halfway up the sides of the front seats. If two passengers rode in the back portion of the car, they were allowed to look at each other. This became real popular with my sister and I when I achieved the age where

I grew too big to sit between the front seats. The car could seat two people very comfortably in the front seats. The car could also seat one or two people very uncomfortably in the back portion. Seat belts were not available in those days, so bracing yourself for all manners of gyrations was a must.

The Ford coupe had a feature in addition to the starter on the column which allowed manual control of the crankshaft. It could be hand-cranked as a second option if the car failed to start the easy way. On occasion during the winters after I was seven years of age and thereafter, I would need to help my dad by manipulating the starter while Dad turned the crank. Sometimes it took an extended amount of time to complete the process. Sitting in a cold car during this time was not blissful; it could cause one to get "cranky." My dad, however, never seemed to complain while performing the hard part of the operation, so I did not say anything.

As I mentioned earlier, when I was three years of age, on one occasion the car did not start, and the roads were not plowed. My mom, who had asthma, ran out of medicine, and Dad drove our tractor to East Town to get medicine. The weather was very cold and windy. Another time with similar conditions when we needed some groceries, he rode the tractor to church on Sunday and purchased the groceries.

Not wishing to look at or touch your sibling added spice to any ride in the roadster. Longer rides became unbearable the older we got, because the close contact became less and less endearing. My comment, "You smell!"-often uttered without cause-was answered with, "So do you!" The rebuttal to my odor may have had some credence, since I tended to avoid taking care of cleaning portions of my body some days as needed.

A calm "We do not need such talk" comment from my dad ended this type of verbal exchange for a period of time, to be replaced by a kick in the shins. Silence was a must in these encounters, until it got too much for my sister. The endurance level for my sister was based on how long she could get the better of me, which was reduced the older I got. At the moment she had had enough, she would yell, "Mom or Dad, he's kicking me!" "She started it! " was always my retort. My mother would then join in and say, "That is enough out of you two."

"He or she started it!" has been a popular retort for children for ages. My children used this phrase many times when asked to stop misbehaving. I used the "That's enough" phrase but my favorite was to tell the individual who was using this as an excuse to retaliate, "Then you end it"

About 1953 the tomfoolery between my sister and I stopped when traveling. It was replaced with just staring at each other or trying to avoid looking at each other. Then about 1954-55, the fumes and dust particles coming up through holes in the flooring of the vehicle contributed to a foggy atmosphere and hence caused all passengers to have a lethargic calmness. By the time a twelve-mile trip to Southeast Town was completed a dazed look covered our faces when observed by others.

In October 1956, my dad purchased a new 1956 Chevy Bel Air. A close friend of my dad's, who decided to supplement his farming income by working as a car salesman, sold him the car and gave him a great deal. This gentleman was successful because he believed in giving the farmers good deals rather than trying to hustle more money out of them. The Ford/Democrat requirement had relaxed a great deal. Buicks and Oldsmobiles were now fashionable for Republicans. Democrats were now purchasing a variety of automobiles. Nash Ramblers, DeSotos, Studebakers were now being obtained. In addition, Chevrolet dealerships were located in West Town, East Town and Southeast Town, so Chevys were readily available. Oldsmobiles also became popular with my uncle the plumber's family, because his oldest son obtained a job at an auto manufacturing factory in Lansing, Michigan immediately after completing high school. This career move although proved to be financially advantageous to him. Plus he provided excellent bargains for his family with his employee discount.

Not attending additional schooling was not real popular with my mother's family offspring as they encouraged their sons and daughters to attend at least two to four years of college or other educational training. My aunt, his mother, had reaped benefits of an education as per obtaining a teaching certificate.

The advent of television commercials also afforded exposure to different types of vehicles to choose from. Taking a ride in the "Rocket Oldsmobile," seeing "the USA in Your Chevrolet," and being told to "drive the new DeSoto"" (*You Bet Your Life*) were enticements for diverse shopping.

The Bel Air was a godsend. Bench seats allowed for the greatest amount of isolation from my sister; it gave an equally comfortable ride to all passengers; and air quality was not an issue within the auto. Also, there was no more cranking of the crankshaft.

We did have one last expedition with the Ford coupe two months before it bit the dust, or should I say we stopped biting the dust. The trip was taken to teach my sister to drive I of course requested to ride along with my dad and her to kibitz the operation.

Unlike my mom's and dad's sisters and sisters-in-law, all nieces learned to drive. My mother never learned to drive. One of her sisters, the DeKalb salesman's wife, learned to drive. One of my dad's sisters drove. Three sisters-in-law drove.

My sister asked my dad, "Why does HE need to go with us?" Dad answered, "Because he might also learn something." My sister mumbled, "Have him ride in the trunk." "What?" Dad asked. "Nothing," my sister answered. I rode in the seat behind the driver, of course.

My dad drove out to a road that was not traveled much. Manipulating a standard transmission was not a natural process for my sister. My father, thinking she drove a tractor at one time, tried to make a comparison for my sister. The resemblance did not ring true for my sister; a jerky, jerky advancement was the upshot for the mile trek back and forth two times. After the second go-around, I tried to encourage her by saying, " That first gear is not bad, that second gear stinks, but third gear is really good." Both my dad and my sister laughed a bit; a third trek seemed to show some improvement. My dad told my mother that he thought my sister improved because she relaxed on the third attempt. My sister confided in me that my humor did relax her, which was a surprise.

The coupe shifting lever was on the floor; the Bel-Air shift lever bar was on the steering wheel column-same church, different pew. The practice that day and a few times after supported my sister in operating the driver's training car when the time came for her instruction. While driving in the Bel Air, she was free of any stupor she had experienced while driving the Ford.

The car I navigated after obtaining my license was a 1960 Impala. This car was built like a tank. My opportunity to drive this machine did not start out well. Six months after passing the necessary road and written test, I came up to a four-way stop but did not completely stop. I had missed a time for taking a test in English class and had just had a fruitless discussion about making it up with the nun who taught the class. She and I had prior problems, so I was rather upset.

A police officer nearby witnessed my error. I was given a ticket. Being a new driver, I was placed on probation by a judge who wore his glasses very low on his nose and looked at me through his glasses. A lecture and an explanation followed regarding what would happen if I received another ticket, which was the loss of my license for ninety days. This tag would be on me until I was 17 1/2 years of age.

I talked to our high school principal. I plead my case, and she allowed me to make up the test.

The judge scared me enough that I was extra careful when I took to the roadways. My mother would remind me of it each time she rode with me, which about 95 percent of the time. I was not allowed to go to any social functions at any time. The only time I drove solo was to run errands and attend work at a drive-in restaurant.

The probation was administered in May of 1963. In the first week of August, my mother felt sorry for me when I asked her if I could go out to a teen night spot. When I arrived at the dance location, I met up with my two secondcousins, the calf riders. We met three girls from a nearby town southeast of Southeastern Town. They wanted to leave and told us to meet them at a local hamburger hangout. We followed them for several blocks, then they came to a four-way stop. They stopped. I stopped and went. To this day I know I made the proper stop, but a police officer who was down a block from the intersection, making his own turn off a side street, said I did not stop at all. I told the police officer I felt I had stopped properly, but he disagreed. I then told him of my probation and how I was being extra careful. I thought honesty might work; I was desperate. He told me, "Tell that to the judge."

My cousins remained mute about the situation; they did not attest that I did stop. The ticket was provided. I left my cousins off at their car, to a Larry Mondello and Beaver farewell (See you later Beav) On my way home, I believe I heard a bugle playing taps.

The next morning I faced a different type of music: I had to tell my mother of the results of my night out. After some threats of tribulation, I arranged my meeting with the judge, my mom, and me. I charted what I was going to say on my behalf. I was going to tell the judge how the officer could not possibly see that I had not stopped, because a large building blocked his vision. Plus, he was a block down the street turning off a side street, at the time of my approach to the intersection.

The Judge did not give a me chance to say anything; he just looked down his nose through those glasses and said, "Do you understand you have no further options?" I said "Yes, but..." He said, " There are no 'buts', your license is suspended for ninety days. You were warned this would happen, and you did not heed my warning. We will see you in ninety days." My attempt at being a barrister discouraged me from any thoughts of that profession. I "told it to the judge," but he told it to me. I still have problems talking to people when they look at me through their glasses low on their proboscis.

When I first moved to Southeastern Town, one day, I witnessed a girl deliver the local paper. A few days later I asked her if she knew of any paper routes that may be available. As luck would have it, she told me she was giving up her route because she was going to work in her uncle's store, and she had been accepted as one of the junior varsity cheerleaders at our public high school, requiring her to attend practice during the delivery time period. I learned the route after a week; the young lady taught me well.

The first four days of running the route alone went well. Friday was the day to collect for the week's deliveries, unless other arrangements were made by the customer to collect biweekly or monthly. The first Friday of my collection process was going well until I came to a house, where, when I knocked on the door, a man came forth very inebriated. I asked him for the fee. He was ardent, hostile, and threatening. He made comments about young kids not having respect for others, and other uncivil actions of the day's youth. I listened to him for a period of time, not knowing whether to stay and plead my case or leave. I was not accustomed to dealing with a person who was drunk. I finally left.

The next day (Saturday), I was greeted at the door of the man's house by the man's wife and the same gentleman. The man apologized to me. He was contrite. They both explained that their son had been a police officer in a larger municipality. A sixteen-year-old boy killed him when he tried break up a street fight. The one-year anniversary of the date of his death caused the man to drink too much, and he took it out on me, a young man he did not know and had never seen before. The paper subscription fee was forty cents; from that day forward I received fifty cents each week.

I enjoyed working the route. I learned business and management skills early on while dealing with the public. One learning experience was discovering that not everyone pays their bills; some postpone them until you push them a bit. Sometimes looking pitiful helped. I had between seventy-five and eighty customers most of the time. Many of them were retired people, widows, and widowers.

There was a mobile home park on my route. Many of the occupants of the homes were college students. One of the benefits of the route was seeing the young ladies each day. After getting to know the people, I would arrange each day so different people would be my last delivery. That way I could spend some time with them once I delivered all my papers. They all enjoyed the company.

The worst part of the job was stopping deliveries for people who failed to pay you. I charged one lady twenty-five cents a week because she was a widow who did not have much money, and reading the paper was her life. She gave me a birthday card, a Christmas card, and an Easter card which had been given to her previously. She would merely cross out her name and put mine in.

The summer after my dad died in April 1961, I purchased a bicycle with money I had banked from various sources. This was my means of transportation for my paper route during the warmer months. Many people were amazed at how I could get off my bike and on so quickly to place the paper where the customer wished it to be deposited. I did not take a long time to deliver the papers; most of my time on the route was spent visiting with customers.

I had a transistor radio I purchased with my first earnings which I would hold dear to my heart. I placed it the chest pocket of my shirt during the summer months. My clients said they knew I was in the neighborhood when they heard the music or a baseball game on the radio. On warmer days, an orange pop/soda from a cooler was a treat for me prior to the end of my workday. Sometimes a cold refreshment was offered by one of my customers. During the cold months, a cup of hot chocolate was extended.

The bike was my means of transportation to all points that I wanted to go, including school during warmer months. Walking was a means of getting from one point to another during the winter months. School was one and a half mile from home. I trekked to school and back everyday.

One night a friend and I ran home from the school after basketball practice so my sister could give him a ride home to his house three miles out in the country. Ah, to be young again! Walking and biking has always been a good method of keeping in shape. The young lady that I took the route over from and I remained friends. She became homecoming queen at the university in Southeastern Town.

Basketball practice for junior high ball interfered with my paper route, so I had to give it up after a year and a half.

On April 1, prior to the ticket incident, I obtained a job working at a drive-in restaurant. Initially I worked as a carhop. A speaker was available for order transfer to a inner portion of the establishment. The order was then brought out to the car for the customer. This made for some fun for my friends. Many came in for this specific purpose.

Words like "Sweetheart," "Lovie," "Honey," "Honey bun," "Sweetie," "Sweetness," and "Dear," preempted or were used throughout the order. I was the only boy among girls, which had its benefits. When one of these girls answered the speaker unit my friends would say " Send that long-legged sweetheart of a boy out with our order." Although I always could take a joke, when I moved inside to assist in cooking, I was relieved that that sort of humor ended.

The restaurant was two miles from our home, so when I lost my license, my bicycle became necessary again. The chain needed upgrading, and a tire needed replacing. The first time I received a ticket, my mom took pity on me and had my sister give me a ride to work when she could. After the second ticket, I was on my own for transportation.

Riding bike, although adequate during my earlier years for travel and keeping in shape, was no longer "cool" after obtaining your license. Bike riding was replaced by "cruising" with a car once you became a operator of an automobile. Walking became my preferred method of getting from place to place after my peers indicated my breech of etiquette when they saw me riding my bicycle. Bringing up my loss of license was not option, since it only caused possible added embarrassment. The money spent on repairs of the two-wheeler was fruitless since I had to sneak around when I did ride the bike. Taking streets where I would not be seen made most trips longer, so the bike soon went back into storage. Walking was found acceptable if I could not find a ride. When the ninety days were up, I had more than one reason to be, happy to be traversing the roads again as the driver of "the tank." No tickets were given to me the remaining portion of my high school days.

I worked hard for the restaurant owner, who was a taskmaster. If we were slow, he would find things for me to do. A number of times he would take me over to his home, and I would perform a variety of yard work for him. When I had basketball practice, I asked the owner if I could be scheduled to not work during the time I had practice. He declined and said, "You work my hours."

I left the position and took a job working at a woman's clothing store cleaning the store and performing other odd jobs that the manager requested.

Once or twice a week I saw the district manager who had hired me. I worked a few weekends moving clothing from one store to another in different towns and cities with him.

A fire started in a restaurant and burned the food establishment and one of our stores in another town forty-five miles west of Southeast Town. (This was the town where I obtained my college education later on.) I basically worked retaining all the clothing that had not burned and any equipment we could save. I spent four days from eight o'clock in the morning until six or seven each evening working.

The district manager had the clothes dry-cleaned and sold them with a sale price tag on them; however, the price was the original cost of the item prior to the fire. No mention was made of the items going through a fire. Surprisingly, he sold all but a few items. He said to me, "A sucker is born every minute." I questioned his credibility. I told him I believed it was false representation. He said it was just a trick in marketing, and that I should keep it to myself and learn something from it.

We were close enough that he offered to sell me a 1956 Triumph, an English sports car that needed a lot of work, for a good price. He said he would help me fix it up. I asked my mom if I could make the purchase. My mom put the kibosh on that quickly, something about saving my money for higher education. Plus it was not American or Democratic or even Republican to own the auto.

One day when I came to work after about a year of being employed, I was told by the district manager not to come down in the basement of the store where the manager had her office for a while. He said he and the manager would be in conference.

The basement had supplies for the store. We ran out of boxes which clothing was placed in at the time of purchase. I needed to get some boxes, so I went down to get some. When I approached the office, I saw the district manager and the manager in a compromising position. I sort of ignored what I saw and retrieved the boxes.

Both individuals were married, and the couples saw each other socially. Although this was my first exposure to an affair, I had reason to believe something was going on prior to this by seeing the actions of the two when together.

The next day when I reported to work, the district manager met with me before I began my routine work duties. He said his boss was performing a quality control inspection and said I was not doing my job well enough and informed him to fire me. I was probably doing a better job than I ever had. I had never heard hide nor hair of this man before, and I still had not seen this mystery man, as supposedly he had left the district manager to do his so-called bidding.

My belief was that there was no quality control boss, and my witness of the incident the day before caused the need for me to be removed from the premises. I had thoughts of extortion for a minute, but rational motivation stopped me and I said, "Okay, thank you for the time you employed me." This was the only time I was ever fired from a job. Looking back on the ordeal with the "smokescreen" of the clothing and the affair, I was glad I did not "triumph" over my mother regarding the purchase of the vehicle from the district manager. I did get good references later life in from both the restaurant owner and the district manager.

Soon thereafter, I started working for my uncle, who was the custodian at our school. I helped him clean the church and school on special occasions and helped him shovel snow at various locations around the convent, priest's residence, church, and school.

Many mornings I had to get up before the streets and roads were plowed to take the mile-and-a-half trip to the site. Some mornings I went where no man or machine had gone before with the "Impala Tank." Nothing ever stopped us from making it through to our appointed purpose.

One Saturday night, the roads were a little slippery when I was coming home from a night out at a dance. I failed to negotiate a right turn one block from our home. The "Tank" slid and bent a street sign to a sixty-degree angle. I expected a great deal of damage to the vehicle; however, when I checked for damages, I found only a small nick in the license plate.

The next morning when we went to church, my sister was driving. My mother said, "Oh look, someone must have run into that street sign and bent it over." I said, "Yes, they did," with no further remarks.

A bicycle came back into my life as a recreational and exercise vehicle during my college days and after I was married. A ride on a bike has always been serene when alone or with others. Riding a stationary unit has become fashionable for exercise, but the scenery is much better riding in the fresh air with a regular two-wheeler.

My wife and I rented a bicycle built for two once, and we took our oldest daughter, who was almost two, with us. She rode in a child's seat, and she fell asleep near the end of the ride.

I taught bicycle safety for two years through the county 4-H program in 1984 and 1985. (4-H stands for: Hands, Health, Heart, and Head and the slogan is: "Learn by doing," or sometimes noted as "Learn to do by doing." Most of the learning and education is through hands-on experience by the youth.)

We took a field trip to McDonald's each year which was located in a village ten miles east of the town we lived in. I had about eight to ten young boys and girls in the class each year, and we took the back roads to our destination. A friend of mine followed behind us in a car for safety and additional supervision. The trek was educational and rewarding for my friend, the kids, and me.

Both years I did not want the kids to feel I could not keep up with them riding, so I pushed myself to the brink, not taking rests too often. I would only stop when the kids said something about taking a break. Years later I heard from the participants through my kids. They said to them, "Your dad sure pressed us on. We wanted to stop a few more times than we did; we had trouble keeping up with him." I was sore for days after our adventure, so the pain was the result of my vanity. I have continued over the years to ride a bike for recreational purposes and exercise.

The only passenger train ride I ever took was in May of 2008 on the way back from a Chicago Cubs game to our home in southwestern Michigan. A buddy of mine and I took a different train ride once when we were in high school.

A freight train that passed through Southeastern town made three to four stops most days. My pal and I decided to jump on an empty car at the first stop on the north end of town. It was our plan to get off at any of stops that followed. Best-laid plans of mice and men, the train stopped at a location where we would be easily observed. We decided to continue to ride the rails to a spot less conspicuous. Unfortunately, the next stop did not occur until ten miles down the road. We did get off the train unnoticed however, we had to call my buddy's mother to come pick us up. The trip was exciting but tense also, as we did not know what might be in our future minute-to-minute.

My friend's mom and my mom did not travel in the same circles, so I took a chance and did not tell my mom of our excursion. My mom never found out about the day my buddy and I played hobo and rode the boxcars. I did have a couple close shaves a couple years later when my buddy's mom made a comment in passing, but my mom did not catch on, or did know about the event and chose not to go there. My buddy and I never really knew.

I have had a few interesting Greyhound bus rides. It seems the longer the expected trip or ride, the more in depth conversation that occurs for you and the person who sits beside you. I had a trip from Detroit to Southeastern Town in 1967, a three-hour trip with several stops along the way. A man who sat beside me never stopped talking to me from the time we boarded to our final destination. Most of the chatter appeared to be a mess of bull. I had just broken up with my girlfriend whom I had just visited, so I was not interested in communicating with him. My lack of response did not stop him from continuing his prolonged discourse. One the tales he told that stuck with me was that he dated Ann Sothern who had some popularity on television at the time but more so during the 1950s and earlier in the movies. He said he grew up with her in Valley City, North Dakota, and her last name was Lake. I wrote off this tale and others he told as the product of a man that knew he would not see me again, so anything was open season. The man looked like he had been rode hard and put away wet a few times and appeared down on his luck, so I further envisioned that he was full of baloney.

Years later I was looking through a book on Hollywood stars and discovered that Ann Southern was born in Valley City, North Dakota, and indeed her birth name was Harriette Lake. Maybe he was part of her life.

I had a few more similar trips on buses. I did have a trip of some length where a girl close to my age sat beside me and did not say a word. My appearance must have turned her off; she was shy; or she did not wish to listen to another's life story or speak of her life story. Some trips were engaging and enjoyable. It helped pass the time when equal time was spent listening and conversing.

I only graced the seat of a motorcycle once, or should I say I lacked grace when the opportunity arose. I rode my future brother-in-law's Honda when I first dated my wife. I lost control twice riding at a moderate speed. The experience swore me off ever operating a motorcycle or riding one with another person.

I have taken a few short boat trips, but never a cruise. The only cruising I ever did was during my high school days in a car looking for girls to talk with, but once I met up with them I failed sometimes to put words together, especially with someone I found interesting and attractive. I am sure it is a very rewarding recreational opportunity and a fuel-saving means of transportation, but I just never had the urge to saddle up.

Speaking of saddling up, I rode a horse once. A friend of mine from Southwest Town had a horse that was trained to stop when you let loose of the reins and would go faster the more you pulled on the reins; however, my friend and his brothers failed to mention this when I saddled up. The culprits just told me to touch the horse with my heels a bit, and the horse would go. I did this, and the horse began to trot a little and then moved at a good, comfortable pace down the road from my friend's home. Everything was going well until after about a half a mile down the road, I pulled on the reins to have the horse turn around and head back from whence I came. The horse instead started to quicken its step, and the more pressure I gave the reins, the faster he went. Just as I was about to fall off the horse, I grabbed the horse by the neck; by doing so, the reins were released, and horse stopped. Not being ready to brace myself, I went flying off the horse onto the gravel road.

A few moments, later my buddy's brother came to rescue me. He explained to me that the horse was my friend's horse. My friend had had polio as a young child, so the horse was trained differently. My friend did not have a lot of strength in his hands, but he did in his arms from wheelchairs and crutches. This sounded logical.

My friend's brother guided me back to the house with the proper handling procedures. When I returned to my friends house, he and his brothers were laughing and made some cracks like "Ride 'em Cowboy." I rode the horse a few more times during my visit.

I never again had an opportunity to ride an equine. I thought about it many times but just did not have a chance to do so. I have always loved horses, though. I have gone on sleigh rides and hayrides drawn by horses.

The snowmobile is a vehicle that many people use for recreation but also is used in some parts as transportation and in emergency situations. I never owned one but have ridden on some with friends a few times.

My uncle who was my sponsor developed Alzheimer's when he reached the age of eighty years old. He endured the condition during the 1990s. It was difficult to see him a pillar of his community, go through the malady. One time I visited him and my aunt, who was unparalleled in her care for my uncle. I was visiting my aunt, and my uncle was sort of mulling about. After about an hour or so I noticed that my cousins, who were the sons of the township supervisor, were across the road working on a snowmobile, trying to get the machine started. I periodically glanced over to the area where they were laboring. After a bit they caught the eye of my uncle. Although my uncle no longer was allowed to operate a tractor or a car, he did go for supervised walks. My aunt suggested that my uncle and I might go over and see what the boys were up to. So my uncle and I proceeded to trek on over to the site.

We stood there for a few minutes observing the action. My cousins said they had checked about everything. Finally my uncle asked them whether they had checked the fuel. The boys mumbled a little and than checked the unit indeed, the machine was out of gas. As soon as they added the fuel, the snowmobile purred. My uncle said glibly, "You just never know." My cousins and I just shook our heads and chuckled.

Hitchhiking was a good mode of getting from one place to another when I was in college. This method would get me from Southeast Town to the college town west of my home, where I attended for higher education, and back home. I met many different individuals, and it was a learning experience meeting these people with diverse personalities from different walks of life.

A mother and daughter picked me up in a Lincoln Continental, my only ride to this day in such a treasured property. Many other luxury cars have come along, but the Lincoln has always been my prized vehicle of choice. The company was great; the mother and daughter were really attractive. The daughter was close to my age. This was when eight-track tapes first came out, and they had an eight-track player in their car. So I sat back, relaxed, and listened to Johnny Rivers and the Four Seasons, with occasional sharing of thoughts. For a farm boy and small town boy, it was hog heaven.

Another time a man picked me up in a Model A convertible. It took almost two hours to take a one-hour trip, but the man warned me. It was a nice day full of sunshine with just the right temperatures, so I really enjoyed the ride.

It took a friend and me ten rides to take the road back to college from Southeast Town. The words of the day were, "I am just going a little ways, but you're welcome to ride with me. " The individuals were mostly farmers going from one small town you passed through to the next . One day my friend and I were walking on campus. Two girls we knew from a class we all had together asked us if they could walk with us. My friend said, "We're just going a little ways but you're welcome to walk with us," and we snickered a bit. They looked at us rather oddly so I explained the joke to them. I guess they understood; however, they did not appear to see our humor. I guess it was one those situations where you had to be there and go through it to see the comedy.

I received a ride in a Triumph convertible as nighttime had set in. I experienced going around a curve at sixty miles an hour in a low rider.

I obtained a ride with some young kids a short distance. The driver drove at high speeds, taking curves very sharply. One of the boys said, "Don't mind him; he just got his license." They were either messing with me, or the kid really had some problems with a lead foot.

A truck driver gave me a ride once, the only time I ever rode in a big rig. He was hauling steel. He was quite amusing, as I remember. He was an older man, and I remember him telling me he was driving part-time. He said he was semi-retired, then gave me a coy look to see if I understood his pun. He told me he had hauled steel for many years, and so other truckers called him " the steel-driving man," akin to John Henry, the railroad builder

I met many, many nice people while hitchhiking. In those days, it was a much safer means of getting from college to home and back, or to other places, for students.

Presently the practice of hitchhiking and picking up the hitchhiker has become almost obsolete, mostly because of questionable security for both parties. Times have changed, though, and most students now have their own vehicles.

Nine months after my mother passed away in 1967, I purchased my first car. The car was a Chevy Biscayne. This car transported me on several dates. It was the location for a break-up by a steady girlfriend, prior to my meeting my wife, and was the location for me to ask my wife to marry me.

My wife and I were married on August 30, 1969. We went on our honeymoon in the Biscayne. We brought our first child home from the hospital in the Biscayne.

My wife ran over my leg with the Biscayne.

My wife and I were taking our firstborn daughter who was born June 8, 1970, to have my wife's sister babysit her. Our daughter was about eighteen months old. My wife had to go to her job; she worked at a supermarket. I needed to attend my college classes. It was a typical winter day for northwestern Michigan. It had snowed about three to four inches, covering an icy surface below for road conditions.

I attempted to drive up a steep hill that we needed to negotiate to get to my sister-in-law's house. There was a drop-off of considerable depth on each side of the road. I made it up the hill about halfway, when we began to slide sideways. The car straightened out a bit when I backed up but began to slide again soon after. I put the car in park, got out, and had my wife take the wheel. I than asked her to back up, and I intended to guide the car down the hill manually. This went well for the most of the backward journey downward, until I slipped and my upper ankle went under the wheel of the car.

The snow actually created a shock absorber. We managed to get the rest of the way down the hill once I gathered myself. Nothing was broken. I did have some bruising, and I was lame for two or three days.

My mother-in-law became an emergency last-minute babysitter.

My wife took some ribbing for some time until about six weeks later. She went grocery shopping and was placing the groceries in the car when she caught the corner of the car door with the area just above her eyebrow. The result was a black eye. Those who knew of the tire-over-ankle incident said, "Oh, he got you back." My wife told them many times what had happened, but the ribbing still prevailed for both of us.

My wife, daughter, and I went through college life from September 1970 to March 1973. The mobile home park we lived in before I took a job in 1973 was about a half mile from campus. We had a woman babysit for us who lived in married housing approximately the same distance from our mobile home. The day of the ankle-tire-incident, she could not babysit.

Normally every day after I completed my classes, I would pick up my daughter from the babysitter and have her ride on my shoulders. She would straddle my neck, and I had a makeshift cloth belt which I placed around her back and around my forehead to keep her in check. I would carry her diaper bag in one arm and my books in the other arm. We would walk over hill and dale in this manner.

Well, one particular day when we were walking home, she fell asleep about a quarter of the way home. Then a minute or so later, she pooped her pants. What a treat I had trying to keep my daughter balanced-who was basically dead weight on my shoulders-carry my books, carry my daughter's diaper bag, and smelling a freshly made bowel movement. It quickened my step a bit; the arrival home could not happen too soon. Love for a child comes to fruition when something like that occurs.

The Biscayne took me to a number of interviews and our mobile home the day we moved the unit 108 miles to the county where my first full-time position in the health field took me.

I remember it well. It was March 29, 1973. The company that was going to move the unit arrived at 10:30 a.m. instead of 9:00 a.m. When they proceeded to pull the unit off the lot, one of the tires went flat. This caused a delay until 12:30 p.m. before the tire was fixed, and we were ready to go.

There was a 3:00 p.m. curfew for pulling any units through the county just before the county where our mobile home was to be located. We had to pass through two larger municipalities on the way also, one before the county in question, and one in that county.

My wife and I watched our home bounce down the highway at average speeds of sixty and sixty-five miles per hour where the driver could maintain these speeds. A few times the wheels went off the road a bit. Our thirty-two-month old daughter sat in the back seat and said, "Look, wheels off" when this occurred. My confidence level that we would still have a place to live at the end of the trip was tested.

We made it through the county in question at 2:45 p.m. Another thirty minutes later, we arrived at the site.

The company driver chuckled that he had his copilot check the insurance policy in the glove compartment a few times during the ride for coverage if the mobile home turned over. Some time after the journey I could look back and smile, but the idea of his humor was defective at the time. In one way I was thankful we did not get fined, and we made our final destination. In another way, I was unhinged thinking of what could have happened. My wife told me to lighten up. So I took the high road and thanked both men for getting the unit delivered safely, using the term loosely.

When we unpacked our possessions that we had boxed up for the ride, amazingly nothing was broken. A clock did come up missing that had metal bars coming off from it like sunrays. It was never found. I told my wife the mobile home lived to see another day, but the clock's time ran out.

The Biscayne served me well, but in the fall of 1973 I decided to trade her in for a different vehicle. A 1973 Vega was her replacement. It proved to be prophetic as OPEC (Organization Of the Petroleum Exporting Countries.) created an oil embargo on oil products in October 1973 as a result of the Yom Kippur War (Arab-Israeli War). The Biscayne and the Impala Tank were therefore not popular anymore. I was told several times after my purchase that the engine would blow up somewhere around seventy thousand miles.

In 1975 the rustproofing I had been talked into by the dealership failed to hold up. The company basically told me, "So sad, too bad;" the dealership should not have rustproofed a Vega, as the body could not be guaranteed. Needless to say, I removed that dealership from places to shop after some bothersome discussion with all involved, even some top dogs who said I was barking up the wrong tree.

I became real familiar with Bondo Putty filler. I placed this substance in several areas of the car. A friend of mine who was a good old boy from Arkansas and one of the nicest guys you could ever meet gave me advice. He was a mechanic but from time to time had worked in some body shops. After my application of Bondo and the necessary sandpapering, my friend painted the vehicle. The original color was white, but I painted the auto yellow my wife's favorite color.

The car took us on a trip to Georgia in 1976 to visit my wife's sister's family. We got lost, partly because of a detour in Charleston, West Virginia, on this trip.

It was in West Virginia that I learned that a "far piece" was somewhere between ten, thirty, and seventy miles. When I asked a man for directions to the main highway he gave the far piece part of the directions. A second gentleman, after I had traveled thirty miles told me of the far piece again with the same roads to travel. A third gentleman, after another thirty miles were achieved, again told me of the far piece with the same route. Ten more miles after the third stop provided the highway we needed to be taking.

This trip also introduced us to a last-chance motel that provided a six-inch-circumference fan for cooling off the room on a very hot night. Green water was available from the showerhead and other faucets. A trip to a Big Boy Restaurant in the same location also included an embarrassing moment caused by my oldest daughter, when she grabbed a small U.S. flag out of the centerpiece on the table and sang "I'm a Yankee Doodle Dandy." Several customers and the staff of the restaurant looked like they were going to stare a hole through us.

Rust again overtook the auto in 1978. It had sixty-nine thousand miles on it, so I never knew whether it would blow up at seventy thousand miles.

In 1977 I was talked into buying another Vega, a red unit. With proper maintenance and oil changes, the car provided one hundred five thousand miles of service to my family and me.

In 1985 I purchased a green 1978 Ford station wagon which had a rear door that could either be opened sideways or dropped down, depending on which latch you operated. There were three bench seats. The back seat could either face backward or toward the front. The seat also would retract along with the second seat so you could have a flat surface to haul things. My kids called it the "Booger Mobile."

The Booger Mobile was used for all types of functions, from hauling items to transporting kids to softball (I was coach), to transporting kids to social functions such as roller skating parties and dance lessons, and for my work duties.

One night when camping out in a tent, it served as a harbor during a violent thunderstorm and short-term sleeping accommodation for the night (Mother and Dad in front seat, and three daughters in retracted-seat area.)

During the years we owned the buggy, our kids said they were embarrassed by the green Booger Mobile. The one and only car they mention when talking about the adventures they had is that vehicle.

I purchased a 1972 GMC short-bed pickup in 1987 from a coworker. The truck had a cap on it and worked well for the tools I carried for my work (augers and measuring devices). It was the first pickup I ever owned, kept me in touch with my manhood, and replaced the Booger Mobile for hauling, as by this time the back door was not working too efficiently.

I discovered after I bought the vehicle that it was similar to a Vega station wagon I had bought for work in 1980. You filled the oil and checked the gas. The gas line sprang a leak right above the exhaust pipe. I made an appointment with a garage five miles from our house to have it repaired. I wrapped a dry rag around the line and headed for the garage without dillydallying around, to arrive as quickly as possible. The garage was adjacent to a gas station. When I arrived, a mechanic came out, smoking a cigarette, and looked under the truck, taking very few precautions to stay his distance from the gas leak. He said "Yup, ya' got a leak there all right; we can fix her right up there. I got a couple things there before ya; we'll get her done as quick as we can." I slowly backed away as he was talking, as far as possible while still able to hear him. I said okay. Just then the guy who came to pick me up to return to work arrived I jumped in the car. I said to my ride, "Let's get the hell out of here before that guy blows up the whole town."

I kept waiting back at work to hear of a major explosion, but picked the vehicle up three hours later without any casualties.

About three months later in the middle of performing a number of services, as I was turning a corner the wheel on the front passenger side came flying off. It rolled about one hundred feet into a open field. After

I gathered myself, I walked out to retrieve the wheel. As I was carrying it back, a friend of mine saw my plight and stopped to lend a hand. As he approached me, I said, "You picked a fine time to leave me, Loose Wheel, four more appointments, and you end up in a field."

My buddy said, "Only you would come up with something like that." Humor sometimes substitutes for nervous reactions. I called a tow truck, and the truck was towed to our home. I never drove it again. I sold it to man I knew who said he thought he could fix it up. He placed a new motor in it and drove it for two more years. The truck was mostly bad luck for me.

I owned several vehicles following the Biscayne which served their purpose for work and pleasure. The last new vehicle was the 1977 Vega (used cars were our only option when bringing up three children) until 1996, when I purchased a new Geo Metro to save money on gas during the years my daughters attended college. A six-foot-four and three hundred-pound man was a sight for others to chuckle at when they saw me get in and out of it and when they saw me drive it. They said I was like Fred Flintstone; instead of pressing the brakes they said I opened the door and stuck out my foot.

My father-in-law called it the wash machine. Early one morning when we were visiting my in-laws, I left to get something, and my father-in-law was still in bed. When I returned, he was drinking coffee. He said, " I heard you start the wash machine this morning."

I have purchased all new vehicles since then, but they have been much more comfortable.

My first plane ride was scheduled six months ahead of time for a Thanksgiving visit to my youngest daughter in 2001 in Virginia. Nine eleven happened and a plane crashed in early November-not exactly a good lead into my virgin voyage in the air. The trip went smoothly, though. I have flown a few times since with no troubles, but I still would rather travel on ground. Claustrophobia appears to be the culprit. Although I have ridden in a few taxicabs in Chicago and San Francisco, the airplane, I must admit, is much less pressure packed.

A minister ran off the road into a ditch. Another man came along and asked if he was all right. The minister said, "Yes, the Lord's riding with me." The other man said, "You better let him ride with me; you're going to kill him."

# TALE TWENTY-THREE

# Food Services or Health Services: That is the Question

MY HIGH SCHOOL COUNSELOR ADVISED me to never take any advanced science classes or advanced math classes in college if I was accepted to any college I applied to in the fall of 1965. (I did not set the world of education on fire my first three years of high school.) My application to the college in Southeastern Town was not accepted. My application for the college west of my home was accepted with probation for the summer term 1966. The grades I provided for both schools to review were bizarre. I enrolled in a general education program at the western school.

My summer term was filled with a variety of happenings. My roommate in the dormitory I stayed in was enrolled in a technological program, so he did not have much out-of-classroom work and reading. So my studying was pretty much done in the library or in a corner of the dormitory lounge.

My roommate wanted to introduce me to a girl from his hometown who was supposed to be" easy". She was visiting the campus for a day-and-a-half orientation. I prayed to the Lord the night before I was supposed to meet her and her friend (who was supposed to be equally promiscuous) to have something happen that we would not meet them.

I did not want to act like I was not "a man of the world," like my roommate projected he was, but my morals also haunted me.

The evening came and I indeed was introduced to "the girl" and her friend. She was a wonderful girl, and so was her friend. We went to a local college hangout, drove around campus in her car, and really had a good time.

When we got back to the dorm, my roommate said, "Oh, they must not have been in the mood." I told him he was a jerk for speaking of the girls in the manner he did. This did not set well with him. He said " You calling me a liar?" I said, "Yes, I am". He said, "You are a f---head," and took a swing at me. I grabbed his arm and put it behind him and told him to settle down.

We did not talk much after that. He only came to the room to sleep and bathe, and he spent the rest of the time with some other students in his program. This was fine with me because prior to our falling out, he never stopped talking. After our episode, I believed, most of it was a mess of bull. According to him, he had been about everywhere, seen everything, and done everything. His absence from our room allowed me to study in the comfort of my room.

I will admit he was a blessing my first few nights in the dorm. I had never been away from home before, and the first couple nights his chatter helped get my mind off being homesick. He was tolerable those first few days because he spoke of his family, so I think he was a bit homesick also.

When I looked back at the "easy girls" incident, I kicked myself for falling for his story. I should have known better.

My cousin, who was a Green Beret, was killed in Vietnam also that summer. He was a mountain of a man, was ten years older than I, and was my hero before his death. He ran a milk route when he first got out of high school. He could lift two full milk cans into a truck at the same time. He played right guard in college football for the college in Southeastern Town. The Green Bay Packers scouted him in 1961.

A gentleman who ended up being my best man in my wedding (as well as my oldest daughter's godfather) and I took a trip to his dentist in a city forty miles south of the college. He had obtained a special permit to drive his parents' car for a week on campus. We got up at 6:00 a.m. to be at his appointment at 7:30 a.m. We were then going to head home to Southeastern Town an eight-five-mile trip home. My friend had a cleft palate, so he had to go to a special dentist in this city.

I was introduced to homeless individuals as we witnessed men and women coming out from areas where they had been sleeping for the night. This was my first exposure; we discussed their plight with sadness .

We arrived early, and 7:30 a.m. rolled around to no avail. The dentist did not show. Minutes turned into a half hour, then into forty-five minutes. Finally my friend checked the appointment card. He then discovered that the appointment was for a year prior, same day, same time, different year. We proceeded to head home to Southeastern Town, both sleepy.

It was a nice trip, new territory for me to observe, and nice scenery. I commented to my comrade that I was enjoying the ride and that if he wished someone to accompany him to a bogus appointment again, I would be available; only could we take a different route so I would see other parts of Michigan. The middle finger was extended by the driver.

Once we arrived at my house, I said, "Thanks for the buggy ride, and remember my offer." He just rolled his eyes. I brought it up few times after that too. He found a little more humor as time went on.

A professor who taught a sociology class came in and lectured for half the session with his fly wide open and part of the bottom of his shirt sticking out through the zipper. When he looked down and discovered his error, he calmly tucked the shirt in, zipped up his pants, and continued to lecture without missing a beat.

We had a biology class in an auditorium with theater seats at 7:25 a.m. I had been studying two nights late in a row for two tests. Some time after our lecturer began, I fell asleep. I awoke with my head on the shoulder of a girl next to me. We both had attended this class for half the term and sat beside each other every session by this time. I never received much more than a grunt from this girl when I said hello to her. She was a very attractive girl. She never said a word to me after I lifted my head or thereafter. I thank the Lord that I did not drool. I did not fall asleep again thereafter.

I had a history professor who wore striped shirts and checkered pants every day that looked like he slept in them. He once asked a question on a test: "Who killed Cock Robin?" True or false. One day when it was pouring rain, he was down on all fours on the sidewalk, pushing and playing with an earthworm.

My English professor told a student who was having a seizure in class to quiet down, prior to realizing what was happening to the young man. The teacher was suspended for the remaining portion of the term for not reacting quickly to aid the poor fellow. He was replaced with a lady professor who was a sight for a young college boy's eyes. The male students' attendance spiked when she became our mentor.

I had some stressful times before and after tests. I also had a few similar days after the term was over. Two weeks after my last test, I received my grades. A 2.8 grade point average took me off probation.

My high school counselor asked me to see her. She informed me that she had submitted my high school grades again to the college in Southeastern Town including my grades from my senior year. As aforementioned, the world of education was not a high priority my first three years of high school-social life was more important-but my senior year I placed my mind on my subjects.

The upshot was that I was accepted to the college in Southeastern Town. I, however, decided to continue my education at the college where I was presently enrolled.

The first day I was home I went to the A & P store to pick up some groceries. The store was right across the street from the courthouse and other government offices. The Greyhound bus stopped in front of this area and was a spot for other transactions, such as being transported to Selective Services physicals.

As I was exiting the store, I met up with a classmate of mine from Southwest Town, dressed in his army uniform. He said he was on his way to Vietnam; he was just home to visit his family prior to fulfilling his orders. I waited with him until the bus came to pick him up. We discussed his concerns with combat and he said he was ready to do what he had to do. I got him off the subject a bit by discussing getting together when he finished his duties. I wished him Godspeed and shook hands with him as he boarded the bus.

This was a Friday. On Thursday of the following week, the headlines of the local paper announced that he had been killed. The details were not clear, but it was known that he was only at the site of his death for less than thirty-six hours. I never learned what happened. I was shocked, to say the least. Our conversation prior to his deployment still lingers in my mind.

Another bizarre twist is that his brother was a scout in the Marines and was in Vietnam for eighteen months.

I returned to school in September 1966. I was placed in a different dormitory with some interesting characters as roommates, who came from the suburbs of Detroit. From these boys I learned about short-sheeting a bed, water fights, food fights, and growing up near Detroit.

One of the fellows was pretty much a professional student; he was beginning his fourth year in college and was not close to graduation. He had been enrolled in several programs starting with pharmacy and different business programs, and was presently enrolled in a food service management program. His father was a high-muck-a-muck in Detroit Edison, and he was an only child. He was a nice guy, and so were his parents.

My roommate who had the lower bunk in my room was a biology major. He was a baffling character. He talked of living until you were two hundred years old or more with advancement and other progress he thought would occur as a result of biological discoveries he learned from his studies, but he never cracked a book. He ended up flunking out by the next term. In other words, he talked a good line but did not produce grades. My other roommate who shared the room with the Edison fellow majored in business. He was a hardworking student

He was a hard sleeper. One night he told me to wake him up for class the next morning. I woke up and went in to wake him. He mumbled around and said he was awake. After I finished my shower and was almost dressed, I went in to check on him. He had rolled over and gone back to sleep. I got him out of bed, got him in the shower, and left. I came back after my classes, and he was pissed at me because he fell back to sleep in the shower and missed his class. I told him to kiss my butt.

He didn't talk to me for a few days, and then he came around again. Many of the young men on our floor had been together the previous year so the floor was a haven for mischief. As result I did not follow up with the grades I should have had. For the summer term, I barely made a 2.0.

Fall term ended two weeks before Christmas. Two days after I arrived home, notification was received that a fellow three years older than I, who was a neighbor of ours when we lived on the farm, had been killed in Vietnam. He was a wonderful guy who always had a smile on his face and always seemed to enjoy life. Everyone enjoyed being around him.

The winter term my money resources were running out, so Edison Man helped me get a job working in the food service unit. I worked in the dish room.

A meal was only served for breakfast and lunch on Sunday, so dinner was on your own. One Sunday we were cleaning up after lunch. One thing led to another and some of my coworkers talked me into going through the conveyor dish machine with the cold water cycle turned on. Our manager never came in on Sundays, so I gave it a shot. Just as I was exiting the unit, our manager walked in. I was given a strong tongue lashing, along with my fellow participants. Liability insurance was also discussed.

My first food fight was a stitch when I joined in one during the fall term of 1966. The enjoyment was not so great when I had to clean up after one as a employee of the food center during the winter term of 1967.

Edison Man talked me into enrolling in Food Service Management after my winter term; however, I ran out money, so I could not return to school until the fall term of 1967 when I earned enough money to return.

My grades were not that wonderful; again, a result of more socializing than attention to studies.

I obtained a job at the college in Southeastern Town on the grounds-keeping crew, and later I worked as a plumber's assistant. Although I was dating a girl steadily at college, I did get to occasionally have conversations with a coed or more while I was working trimming shrubs, tending to grass, and policing trash. These discussions were a benefit of the job. Working on the plumbing crew was even more favorable since I could get even more up close and personal while I was accompanying the plumber, or on my own, addressing a simple job summons. When I was on my own, I was allowed to drive a Cushman three-wheel utility vehicle. It was a treat to whiz around in this unit. It had a little bell on it which I hit when I approached someone to alert them. Most people would laugh or smile when I did this.

I learned at a young age to play a card game called euchre, which has been very popular in the states of Michigan and Wisconsin for many years. I was my mom's partner after my dad died, when we played with my relatives. I was a "boy sent to do a man's job," a term used by players in the game if you do not play a high enough card to win a play of cards.

The first couple of weeks on my grounds-keeper job, I watched four men play this game every lunch break. A mentally challenged man would eat with me at the same table. The table the four men played the card game at was close by the table my friend and I ate at. Then one day, the partner of an older gentleman who played was absent from work. I was asked to sit in. The older man had complained a great deal about his partner's plays, so I was a little skeptical about playing with him; however, he appeared to be satisfied with my playing efforts. In fact, he complimented me a few times.

The next day his partner returned, and the man suggested that we switch off playing as his partner every other game. The man continued to heckle him but continued to compliment me. After two weeks, his partner told him he no longer wanted play with him. I felt bad. Sometimes he played against us when one of the other men were off work.

The older gentleman was really a good guy but had no tolerance for what he thought was bad playing of cards. The mentally challenged fellow was not treated well by the family he stayed with. They received money for him to supposedly buy clothes for him and provide adequate food for him. There was very much evidence that the caretakers were not using the money correctly by the way he was dressed and the lunch he brought. My partner would bring an extra sandwich or something for the less fortunate fellow. I started to do the same.

Edison Guy would get an allowance every term and spend it on clothes and other things. He would run out of money by the end of the term, causing him to work at the food commons. He gave me some of his shirts he no longer wanted; therefore, I gave the unfortunate man some of my old shirts.

My new euchre partner brought an abundance of carrots. He always said they put lead in your pencil.

I visited my girlfriend on weekends by hitchhiking to "my college." Whether I did so or whether I did not, the mentally challenged man would always ask every Friday whether I was going to the Big City to visit my girlfriend. The college town where my college was located was smaller than Southeastern Town. When I returned on Monday, he would ask, "Did you go to the Big City this weekend?" even if I told him I was not going on Friday.

When my girlfriend returned to the Detroit area for the summer, we broke up in late June. He did not understand that and continued to ask me about the Big City, so I continued to keep up the charade.

I was called in for my pre-induction physical at the same time "The Riots" broke out in Detroit in July 1967. The physical was postponed until later in August. You could walk the streets of downtown Detroit and see the destruction without any problems. The sight still remains indelible in my memory.

I returned to school in September 1967. I entered the food service supervision program. I was assigned to the food commons, where I worked the winter term of 1967 to perform hands-on work out of the classroom. I had mended some of the wounds from the conveyor dishwasher incident, but the manager still had some doubts about my commitment to the program. Therefore at times he was extra watchful of my work ethic; he still felt I had vagarious tendencies.

On October 8, 1967, my mother was killed in an automobile accident that my sister, mother and I were involved in. My sister and I recovered from the accident, and I returned to college for the winter term.

I continued to do my fieldwork with the original food manager. He and another manager helped get additional work on campus for me. We had a number of conversations throughout the term, and we got to know each other better .

The program director was a really wonderful lady and a good classroom mentor.

One of my roommates was enrolled in the environmental health program, which was a new program developed by two individuals who had worked in health departments in Michigan and Ohio. There were new laws and codes being developed for the state of Michigan, which would provide the need for staff to be hired to work for local and state health agencies.

I also had a number of friends enrolled in the program. Along the way as part of my curriculum for my program, I took four classes with the members of the health program regarding laws, food safety, and pest control. My interest was piqued a bit, but I continued to follow through with my food service program. Besides, I remembered what my high school counselor had said, never to take advanced math and science classes, and the health program had several of them in the curriculum.

I managed to make it through winter term rather quietly, studying and mourning my mom's death. I received admirable grades. I returned home for time off between terms. My sister and I discussed settling my mom's estate. My sister had taken action in December of 1967 to enter the convent in August 1968. The house was up for sale.

I had met a girl at the Southeastern college during my break, so the spring term brought me back and forth between my college and that college, hitchhiking to visit this girl and discuss further issues with my sister regarding my mother's estate.

Other than the occasional weekend engagement, I had a pretty quiet spring term also. We did have a proceedings one night on an unusually warm night in late April. Panty raids were fashionable in those days, so two dorms near the dormitory I lived in were chosen for this process. I did not participate for two reasons. My old girlfriend was a resident assistant in one dormitory. In addition to that, I no longer was interested in the chase involved.

One of the fellows I spent time with in the dormitory during meals and other times kept talking of not getting caught by the campus security, which could have happened and some retribution handed out. He also made comments about how he was not scared if they did catch him, because he could talk his way out of it. Others and I listened to this for about two weeks straight. Finally on the second Friday night after the raid, another guy and I decided to give the boy a call, indicating we were the campus security.

I called the dormitory floor phone and asked for him. I disguised my voice and told him something similar to this: "We understand that you were present at the panty raid, and we're following up on some leads we received. We would like you to come down to the office on Monday." He was very polite. He said he would cooperate, but he said did not participate. The conversation went on for a little while more with several "yes sirs" and "no sirs" on his part. Finally I used my normal voice and said, " You are a liar, " and both the other guy and I started laughing. He said, "Is that you, Gerry Martin? You jerk!" I said, "It sure is, tough guy, and from now on call me 'Sir' with a capital letter." We rode him hard after that about the raid and my phone call. I told him for some time after that to call me "sir" when he spoke to me.

I performed my spring term co-op with the other food manager, who I worked for in the snack unit he operated in addition to his food commons unit.

Martin Luther King was killed April 4, 1968, and Robert Kennedy June 6, 1968. I had become a casual friend of the soon-to-be president of the Alpha Phi Alpha fraternity as a result of some round table discussions in my 121 Political Science class. During the winter term I learned a great deal about the black man's perspective from this gentleman. This served me well for the rest of my life. He was a very levelheaded young man. I also had a roommate whose father was black and mother was Caucasian. This was not found to be acceptable in those days; therefore, his dad only would bring him to school or pick him up, and they would leave his mother at home in the Detroit-area suburb where they lived. The young man had the features of a black man. I also learned from this young man the hardships of growing up in an interracial home. He did not share this with me until one night a few days after Martin Luther King was killed.

I had a philosophy instructor the spring term who I heard stories about. His residence was in Southeastern Town, where his wife taught college math. He rented two rooms in my college town.

Edison Man told me one story about what three fraternity brothers told of him. He was their adviser, and they went to visit him to discuss a few fraternity issues. They told Edison Man that his rooms were just deplorable with filth everywhere. They said he had two dogs, and while they were there, one of them pooped on the floor. They said he scooped up the poop with his hand (what was hard enough; the rest remained on the carpet) and threw it out the door. He then came back after wiping his hand on a dirty towel, without washing his hands, and continued talking to them. I heard other odd stories about him. I knew he was a little eccentric but found it hard to believe some of the stories. He always appeared to be clean in class.

Then one night during the 1968 spring term, I was hitchhiking home when he picked me up. He had his two dogs in the car. The car reeked of a variety of smells. He was smoking a cigar, or should I say, he was chewing on the cigar. He would open his window and spit some of the cigar out the window, but most of it would run down the outside and inside of the window or down the front of his tie. It was a trip. He would be real somber and then blurt out a question for me. I was really uncomfortable, so I just rode without attempting to ask him any questions or carry on too much of a conversation.

I managed to obtained satisfactory grades again.

The month of June brought the sale of our house and my move to my college town. I rented a one-story apartment in a large house that had been converted into two two-bedroom apartments on the ground level and two apartments upstairs, one of which I inhabited. I shared an outer bathroom/shower and bathtub with the inhabitants of the other apartment.

A friend of mine and his brother rented one of the downstairs apartments. They were both enrolled in the related health program. He and his brother and I discussed the classes they were taking, and I again shied away because of the math and science. They were both attending a couple classes. I was taking the summer off, as none of my classes were available in my program.

The manager who gave me my first job in the food commons and I became very close. He now had a great deal of respect for me being out on my own. He found a couple jobs for me around campus as a way to earn some money.

In mid-July of 1968, the Biscayne entered my life.

One hot summer night with the humidity unbearable and air conditioning absent my friend's brother and I decided to go sleep on the dunes of Lake Michigan, sixty-five miles from our college town. We took nothing but the clothing we were wearing. There are some things you try once in your life and then say, never again; this was one of them. Even though the temperature conditions throughout the area were uncomfortable as per heat, this was not true at about two o'clock in the morning on the dunes. The air off the lake and the surface of the dunes created an unsettling opposite temperature difference, where comfort was now a problem regarding a cold, moist environment, which made dozing off for a short period of time and awakening pretty much the routine for the duration of my sojourn until we left at about 7:00 a.m. My friend's brother said he was not that uncomfortable; however, I told him I could find other ways of having the same kind of fun, like chewing on tin foil or dragging my fingernails down a blackboard.

The Biscayne took me on a few trips that summer to visit my girlfriend (who attended Southeastern college) who lived in the Detroit area. The Detroit Tigers were battling the Baltimore Orioles that summer for the American League pennant. My girlfriend's father did not like Catholics, although he never went to church much; he also hated the Tigers and loved the Baltimore Orioles. Anyone who loved the Tigers was his enemy. He was cordial to me, but he was also combative when he spoke to me. He always seemed to want to argue with me regarding anything I said.

The first time I ever met him, I spoke of the joy I had that my high school had won the state championship in basketball in 1967. I told him it was interesting and pleasant to see guys I played sports with on television in the state finals winning it all. (I could not attend the game because I had final exams.) He commented that Detroit schools beat each other in the tournaments, and then some Catholic school comes to the tournament finals and gets lucky in one game and wins the state championship. (He was a principal at a larger public school.)

I visited my girlfriend on Labor Day weekend in1968. My girlfriend's father was rather capricious when I addressed him directly in conversation.

What had been a fervent relationship for four to five months started to become more warm at this time; I just had not caught on to my girlfriend's signals. The relationship was not strong enough to endure the time intervals between seeing each other during the summer. She did not return to her college until the winter semester. A visit to my campus by her for my college's homecoming in October 68 provided the "I think we should still date each other but we might also start dating other people" statement from her lips. A warm-to-lukewarm relationship developed. Telephone conversations from October to the first week in December just before my birthday were promising one minute and confrontational the next. Any suggestion that I visit her was met with "not right now." The party was essentially over.

On the way home from my Labor Day visit 1968, I decided to take the trip, back through Southeastern Town. I stopped in to visit my second cousin, who had been a person of comfort after my mom died, and her family. She informed me that my friend (would be my best man) had been in an accident with another friend of mine the night before, and they were in the hospital. She also informed me that a friend of mine who lived three blocks from our home in Southeastern Town had been killed in Vietnam six weeks prior. I said, "You are just full of good news."

(The victim of Vietnam, his brother, and others in the neighborhood had played basketball with me at his house every night and day we could during the summer months between our junior and senior year. He was a great guy.)

After we had visited some more, I proceeded to get up to leave. I told her I was going to stop and visit my comrades. She encouraged me to stay and have something to eat. I decided to take her offer.

She and her two teenage daughters commenced making what I thought were a couple pizzas. Now my cousin's family consisted of two sons in college, two daughters in high school, and her husband. With me around the table, there were seven mouths to feed. The boys were exceptional athletes. One of her sons played on the state championship team and held the record for the most rebounds in a career at Southeastern Town college for many years. An eight-inch pizza was presented in front of us that was cut into small pieces. We each had a piece. The eighth piece remained on the platter until everyone had finished their sliver. I expected that another pizza was forthcoming, wrong! The eight-incher was it.

I soon became aware of that when my cousin asked if I wanted the last piece. I said, "if no else wants it, I guess I could find room for it." She said, "You are just like your dad; he could always eat a lot too." I did not take the last piece for fear I might be accused of overeating; besides, some people like pizza for breakfast, and they could have cut it and each have a piece. Breakfast many times has been a smaller meal.

I left and visited my friends in the hospital. They mostly had bruises and facial cuts and were to be discharged the next day.

I developed a friendship the fall term of 1967 prior to the accident with a guy from New York whose father was Jewish and mother was Catholic. He got married over the summer in 1968. When he returned in September, Denny McLain was working on winning thirty-one games.

My friend was a Yankee fan. He rooted against Mr. McLain every time he pitched. We watched together all the games McLain pitched; it added a little spice to our viewing .

This fellow was a real blessing, along with my future best man and my old girlfriend (the R.A.), during the winter and spring terms of 1968 in listening to me while I was mourning my mother's death.

I learned the worth of growing up in a home where a person was exposed both to the Jewish and Catholic faiths. Although this gentleman practiced the Catholic religion, he had a good handle on the proper method of treating others based on both faiths.

His sense of humor was much like mine, so we enjoyed bantering back and forth. He went back to New York after the fall term because his wife did not like the surroundings of the "one-horse town," as she put it. She was a good gal; you had to stay ready for her comments as she could debate with the best of them. We had several discussions on issues of the times. She told me being wrong was my prerogative after we came to a standstill in a discussion.

When the Tigers did win the pennant and the World Series, I was very careful not to bring the subject up in conversation with my friend. I never had any conversations with my girlfriend's dad because I never visited her home again immediately after they won, but I heard from her that he was one of the few people in the Detroit area who were upset that they won. In addition, someone wrote "Tigers World Champs" with a bar of soap on the back window of his car, which I imagine irritated him to no end.

I had a speech teacher in the fall term of 1968 who was a character. If you were late for class or did not complete an assignment, he would get the victim up in front of the classroom to recite the same verse every day. He would say the verse once through with the individual, then the speaker would be required to recite it alone. He would make the person start over if he or she stumbled, until they made it through the verse entirely. The verse was:

Men in the ranks will stay in the ranks. Why?
I will tell you why:
Simply because they have not
The ability to get things done.

I never had to do this exercise, but by the end of the term everyone knew the verse in the class. The professor told us at the end of the term we would always remember the verse. He was right; I can still recite it.

Our class was at 7:25 a.m. There was a portable podium on a desk in the room. Every morning, the first thing he would do was pick the podium up and slam it down and say, "Is everybody awake now?"

He would stop you in the middle of your speech and make you start over if "um" and "a" were ever misused. You learned to pause instead of using "um" and "a" to connect your words in the speech. If you mumbled or did not speak loud enough for everyone to hear, he would yell, "I can't hear you." He clarified the difference between proper and improper hand gestures by lampooning you when you made the wrong body expressions.

I was neighboring an A in the class. Our last day of the term was December 17. I turned twenty-one on December 12. I managed to tip a couple each night thereafter. On December 14, I ran into the speech professor in the bar. I sat and had a couple with him. We discussed some issues. He said I was not a great speaker, but my speeches were sincere, and I appeared to make up for what I lacked in talent with heart and hard work (a left-handed compliment?). I received an A. I was never sure whether the discussion in the bar might have turned the tide.

I was required to take typing as part of my curriculum. I never could type worth beans, maybe for the same reason I could not play any musical instruments. My fingers just don't move with grace.

My instructor, a jolly, big fellow, tried hard to work with me during the fall term of 1968, but I just could not cut the mustard. At the end of the term he asked me if I thought I would be using typing much in my profession. I said I did not feel it would be a very big part of my life in regards to speed requirements; I would be filling out some forms, but that would be the extent of it. He said he felt I probably could plunk my way through that, and he said if I solemnly promised to never say I excelled at typing, he would give me a C in the class. I told him that was a foregone conclusion. He chuckled as he walked away.

One night in the spring of 1968, a large group of black students took over the General Education, Administrative, and Professors' Offices building in a protest movement. They held the building for several hours until the National Guard was called in to remove them. I did not understand at the time exactly what their concerns were. I found out later I was too passive in this regard. I saw the violence end of the concern and not the true reason for the protest, even though I had been exposed to some concerns of the African American through my roommate.

I remember the future president of the black fraternity speaking on a few occasions in our class about our college not advancing past allowing blacks only learning to read. I did not really know what he was referring to. So I asked him for a further explanation. He said that during slavery, blacks were not allowed to read and write, that it was against the law.

I never thought much more about his statements until the fall term of 1968. The black students again took over the college library. This time they only stayed overnight and part of the morning. They exited on their own. I ran into the gentleman who was now president of the Alpha Phi Alpha fraternity, and I asked about the new protest. He sat down with me for a short time and explained that after the first protest it was agreed that the college administration would look into providing more classes that were amiable to the black culture, with language also understandable to the African American. He said they also wished to have black history incorporated into appropriate classes. In addition, they wished to have their social functions recognized by the administration. He said some of their requests were met, but black history was not being addressed for reference in the library, and not enough African American literature, journals, magazines, and periodicals were available in the library. Therefore the library was made the point of protest. He further said their other petitions were not being acted on quickly enough.

I went to the library soon after things calmed down and found, indeed, the library did not have much information as per the black students' needs.

During winter term of 1969, I again investigated whether conditions had improved and found that there was some improvement, but whether it was satisfactory, I did not know. I asked my voice to the black students, and he said there was movement forward, but only time would tell the future. He said it looked more promising than before.

I started to realize that my being friends with African Americans or the information I gathered from them, like I had, could not allow me to fully understand their dilemma. Not even walking a short time in their shoes would help. Forgiving those who trespassed against them must also have been very difficult.

I learned much more about the black man's plight years later when I heard and read about men like Emmett Till, who was killed by two white men for whistling at women, and Medgar Evers who was murdered for standing up for his rights. Generations of unborn learned, have learned, and will learn from the black men and women who lived and died during the period of the late1950s to the early 1970s.

Once the fall term ended, I obtained a job cleaning buildings during the time off between terms with two fellows who were married and in my program.

One of the men worked at a motel as a night clerk from 10:00 p.m. to 6:00 a.m. He said he did not see much action at that time; basically he said it was just watching over the property. He asked me to drop in when he started work and keep him company for a while and maybe play some cards.

I arrived about 9:45 p.m. A young woman who had been working as the day clerk soon began to get her coat and boots on to go home. She said she was going to go home, get her pajamas on, watch a little television, and go to bed. I said, "You might as well, can't dance; one leg is shorter than the other." This was a term I used all the time to say anything you do is okay as long as you have fun doing it. She smiled a bit. My friend and I talked to her a little more, but I noticed my friend acted a little uneasy.

When she left, he said, " Did you not notice when she put her boots on that her one leg was shorter than the other? She had polio when she was young." I said, "Leave it to me to place my whole foot in my mouth. I should have at least had some mustard and ketchup with my shoe leather."

The next day after we completed our work day, my coworkers and I went rabbit hunting . My two buddies told me to circle around, and maybe I could stir up a bunny or two. Unfortunately, we misunderstood each other about the direction I was going, and soon after one of them heard a rustling which was me, but they thought was a rabbit. One of them took aim and fired (to this day I do not know which, they both took the blame) at something they thought was a bunny. The remnants of the shot came about ten feet from my feet. I yelled, "What the H-E double L-L are you doing!" That ended the hunting expedition. Apologies were repeated several times. I said maybe that girl I insulted might like to also have taken a shot at me. My friends said they appreciated my humor but were sorry about what happened.

The next day I arrived at work, my desk clerk friend told me that to his surprise the girl I insulted said I was handsome, seemed like a nice guy, and had a sense of humor. I said, "You are kidding me." My friend knew I was literally crying in my beer regarding my breakup with my girlfriend, so he said, "Maybe this girl might take her off your mind."

I asked her out a couple days later on a Sunday morning. She said she did not feel well and was not feeling good enough to go anywhere. I wanted to go to the movie because I had heard good things about it the title was *The Heart is a Lonely Hunter*. As I was sitting waiting for the movie to start, the girl walked in with two other girls. This built up my ego.

When I returned to work, I told my friend thanks for leading me on. I told him that when I was a junior in high school, two girls set me up and told me another girl wanted to go out with me and that she really liked me. The whole thing was a joke on me. (A year later the girl herself and the two other girls apologized, but I was resentful for awhile.) He said, "No, she actually said that about you." I said, "Sure, I probably ticked her off, and she was just trying to get me back for my comment."

The next day my friend told me that he brought up the movie incident with the girl, and she explained that she had gone out with the same ladies she was with at the movies to someone's house and had a few drinks. She had a stomach ulcer and really had never had any alcohol before, and she had become sick early that Sunday morning. She still was under the weather when I called. Then in the afternoon she felt better, and when her friends called, she decided to go with them.

I spent Christmas 1968 with my friend the food commons manager's family. It was really nice for him to invite me; it was not like having a gathering of your own family, but it was nice. (Thanksgiving that year I had spent by myself in my apartment, which was not so nice.) The manager had a daughter who was four years younger then me. She asked me if I had ever dated any girls from the town the college was in. I explained about the girl who I had recently asked out, but I said I would never marry a "Townie." The people of the college town would call students "Pinheads," and we called them "Townies."

A couple days after Christmas, I asked the girl out again. She accepted and we went to a movie and had a sandwich and a drink after the show.

New Year's Eve was spent with her. She fixed one of her friends up with the fellow who lived in the apartment below mine with his brother. We sat around his apartment and had a few drinks.

We did not go out again, but her friend and my friend went out a few times.

I had managed to get my best grades in regards to point average (3.5) I was winding down with the completion of my two-year degree in Food

Service Supervision and Management. I had to complete winter term and spring term, and I was out of there to face the working world in my chosen profession. The spring term I was only going to have two classes: a 122 Political Science class, and a class regarding management techniques. The winter term classes were all involved with my program major.

The first Friday after the winter term had began in early January, I met a girl at a college dance who was spending her first week in college. I discovered she was eighteen years of age and seemed to be a rather intelligent young woman. We danced some and talked a bit. I walked her back to her dormitory and asked if she would like to go to the show the next night.

The driveway for the house with the four living units extended from the street in front to an alleyway behind the unit. This driveway was rather long, because there was a considerable backyard. My friend, his brother, and I parked in the front area and kept this area shoveled. The couple who lived in the back downstairs unit and the two fellows who rented the other apartment upstairs parked in the back by the alley and maintained an area for their cars to be parked, so there was an area between the two parking areas that had a large snow buildup. You had no other choice but to back up in both directions. The home sat much higher than street level, so there was a bit of a lift to get up to the level area for parking and a sidewalk area that was again a little higher than the street. Therefore, besides shoveling the driveway area, you needed to spend a considerable time clearing this area.

We had considerable snow prior to my date night, so the banks that we created were rather high. We did not overdo the width of the driveway. The level area was appreciable, but near the road we left an area just wide enough to get a car through.

The night of my date, I warmed my car up. My friend's car was parked behind me, so I asked him for his keys to back his car out. After I started his car, I unfortunately did not remove the ice from all his windows. I backed up with his door open to see my way. This worked until I got to the limited width area. The wind caught the door, which caused it to slip out of my hand. I did not grasp the door again until it was too late. My intention was to close the door prior to approaching the limited width area. The door caught the bank and became sprung. Understandably, my efforts to close it were futile.

Several times in my youth I had to admit guilt for a troublesome action, the time I received the two tickets for stop sign neglect being examples. The walk I needed to take in my adult life to tell my friend what I had managed to do was comparable.

There are times when you find out who your true friends are, and your faith in those friends being good people comes to the forefront. My friend said, "Well, I can see how contrite you are. We will work it out."

I called to tell my date that I ran into a snag and would not make the night out.

My friend and I managed to get the door closed enough to drive the car. We took the car down to a service station (in those days service stations were available and were open after 6:00 p.m.) We had to wait a couple hours, but the serviceman did a good job righting the door, leaving only a small fold in the door at the hinge area of the outside of the door.

I met up with the girl the next afternoon at her dorm. We went out for some fries and a drink. She laughed and giggled at anything and everything that was said and done around us, inappropriately at times. She was about six foot one and rather attractive but snorted when she laughed hard. Why I tried to kiss her goodbye at the door of her dorm I have no idea, but I did. She banged her face against mine and giggled. The whole time with her was a train wreck. I think the door incident with my friend's car was an omen and was a sign of the future with this girl.

The next Friday I attended the college dance again and met another girl. One thing led to another, and I asked her if she would like to go to a dance that was being held as part of the winter festival on campus, the next night. She accepted. She seemed to be a nice lady.

Her dorm was near my old dorm, where the dance was, so I walked up to her dorm, leaving my car at home. We walked to the dance. We danced a few dances, then she said she was going to go talk to some guys she knew somehow, and that she would be back. She was gone for about fifteen minutes then she came back, and I asked her if she wanted a drink. I went to get the drink. When I return her guy friends were there talking to her. We danced again and then she went to talk to her "friends" again. This went on for about an hour and a half. I finally told her she was either with me or them. Evidently I was a ticket for her to get to see these guys without being obvious. I left her there and went home.

The following week I met up with those two girls several times. The eighteen-year-old seemed to be following me around, and the other kept asking me to give her another chance. It got to the point that I was hiding out. I thought about trying to go out with the Townie, but my friend told me she had moved and got a job working in the city forty miles south of my college town.

I decided to get out of "Dodge" the following Friday and visit my buds in Southeastern Town for the weekend. I stayed at the lady's house who lived next to our old house in Southeastern Town; she had an extra bedroom and was glad to see me. I did not find anyone to hang out with on that Friday night at the locations I visited. The next night was the same, so I decided to visit the college campus in town. I was sitting down to have a drink when my old girlfriend walked in. She came over, and after some discussion we left and went for a drive. After some further discussion, she indicated she might want to get back together on a steady basis. I said I might also be interested. I dropped her off and kissed her goodnight. The next day I headed back to my college town, as I had a test on Monday.

I told the two girls I had gone back with my old girlfriend when I saw them.

I decided to visit my old girlfriend the next weekend. I arrived Friday night and made arrangements to stay with one of my cousins. I then went to visit her. She came down from her room and informed me that she had a date that night. A heated discussion followed between us. I left angry. I went to my cousins, played euchre, and drank a few brewskies.

I returned to my college town the next day. That night I met a girl who was with some other girls who were dating two friends of mine from the food program. I did not realize at the time that the meeting was setup. We got along pretty good, and she was Catholic, which had been a problem directly with the R.A. lady and indirectly, among other things, with the Southeastern Town lady.

We went out a couple times, and I visited her dorm to study with her for about ten days. Than one night out of the blue she said she was basically going to college to find a man to get married to. I said although I was lonely at times and had no immediate family at my disposal, I was not interested in moving too fast in any relationship.

I ran like a scared rabbit. I now had three girls with a variety of interests in me and one who I had no idea what her interest was.

Valentine's Day rolled around, and I decided to make one last effort with the girl from Southeastern Town college. I sent a bouquet of flowers to her with an apology about showing up unannounced. I received three cards from the ladies of interest. I did not afford them anything in return as I did not want to mislead them, but I must say I had a little high going on (but it was with mixed emotions.) I received no response from the flowers.

One night a couple days after Valentine's Day, I was at the bar when I ran into the desk clerk who had left town. She said she was in town for a day and was thinking about moving back. We talked for some time. She gave me her phone number where she now lived, and she left.

The next week when I was feeling low, I called her. She was cordial, but the conversation was a lot of small talk. Two weeks later, my friend told me she had moved back to my college town.

I decided to go visit her at her house. Her dad and mom were very nice and invited me in. Her dad had said he liked me because I was one of the few guys his daughter ever dated that came in to talk to him and his wife the first time she went out with me. Her sister was also visiting. My desk clerk friend said a few things to me and seemed a bit nervous. She then informed me that she had a date that night. I struck out again. I said, "Okay." However, we still talked some as friends. Her family pretty much told me to stick around and talk. She left for her date and I stayed and washed dishes with her sister. I stayed until I said, "I had better get out of here before she gets home from her date."

Two weeks later I ran into her again. She said she was now working back at the motel as a waitress at the restaurant that was part of the operations, and working catering jobs when they came up. She told me they were looking for some help at times when they had events. One of the classes I had during winter term was learning catering operations. Her boss had visited the campus to put on a few presentations for our class. I went in and talked to him about working, and he said he would call me when he had functions.

I started going in to the restaurant for dinner. We went out a few times and worked together a few times. It was more or less an on-again-off-again relationship until after the first week in April 1969.

We thereafter spent most days together at one time of the day or other. On one occasion we talked until 4:00 a.m. Her dad got up to go to work, and I was still there. He just said, "Hi!" and got ready and left.

I had a 122 Political Science professor during spring term of 1969, who was a chain smoker. I had him for the 121 class, so I knew his habits. We would put a cigarette by his lecture area, and he would cut his lectures short in the 121 class. The 121 class was one hour three days per week, so the class most days lasted forty-five minutes. The 122 class was in the evening from 6:00 p.m. until 7:30 p.m. twice a week. He would let us take a five-minute break in between so he could grab a smoke.

When he came into the class, he would always ask where he left off with his lecture at the last class. Four weeks into the class, some fraternity guys in the class got spring fever and told him he left off where he had begun the previous class. This went on for two weeks. Each lecture was the same, so they would skip out during the break.

I guess he had taught the class for so long he had his notes memorized, plus he was a bit of a nut. I took the class when I did because I had one other class, and that was in the morning, so I had the afternoon to work catering events at the motel/restaurant. I told my now-girlfriend after the second week that we might do something early in the evening if the "boys" decided to play the game again. I told her I would report for attendance and sit in the back and sneak out. The lecture was boring enough, let alone to listen to it again and again. I stuck it out because I was afraid he might catch on some time throughout the class. I told her to wait outside the classroom, and I would meet her when I could sneak out.

Unfortunately the boys agreed the repetition was getting too much, so they decided to give the professor the right information. He started the lecture where he left off the last class. I had sat in the back by one of two doors to the classroom so I could sneak out.

My girlfriend was waiting, so I decided to make a run for it. The girl and I decided to go to a movie; however, just as the movie started, she became ill. I took her home and told her I would check on her the next day.

I decided to go back to my apartment. I sat and read for a bit, then decided to walk up to the dorm that I lived in winter and spring 1968. One of my friends also was in the 122 Political Science class. As I was walking up to the area, I came upon an uprising that involved a group of black students and non-black students. A couple cars were turned over in the student lot. Campus Security and the local police were called in. Unfortunately, I had traveled to the point of no return. A few of the black students surrounded me. Fortunately my Alpha Phi Alpha friend told them I was okay and told them to leave me be. I made a U-turn and headed back whence I came. A few minutes later an officer asked me to accompany three girls to their dorm. One was the girl who played the game at the dance. I never really knew what caused the physical debate.

The ladies thanked me for escorting them. The girl who deserted me at the dance asked me to come in and talk a bit, so I did for a while. Essentially small talk was in order. She said we ought to go out some time. I mentioned I had a girlfriend, but you never know.

The next day I checked on my girlfriend. She said she still did not feel good, and I might need to stay away.

That night I went to the bar in my old stomping grounds (Southeastern Town) with my friend who lived in the lower apartment. He was an excellent pool player, so we played doubles and made a few bucks. I ran into a girl who was in my class in elementary school. We discussed some things we did when we were young.

We had a box lunch event for Valentines when we were in eighth grade (1962). This girl's dad drove our school bus, and we were pretty good friends. I did not have much money to spend because of my dad passing away (1961) and his medical bills still needed paying. My buddies made arrangements with her that my friends and I would bid on the lunch until a certain amount was achieved, then they would allow me to win that bid. She would provide half the money, and I would not look bad. She was still a great gal. Time had not changed her.

Before my friend and I left, I said I might see her again; she said that would be great. We stayed overnight at his grandma's house and returned to our college town the next day.

The third week in May 1969, my girlfriend and I stopped seeing each other as much as we had (almost everyday). I was interviewing for jobs; I had been to Southeastern Town with my friend for a weekend again. We toured some of the bars playing pool and talked to a few ladies.

One day during this period I took a shower in the middle of the afternoon. I always took a pair of pants with me, took my key with me, put something in my door to keep the door from closing, or all three, as the door had a snap lock on it that automatically locked. This day I was in a hurry to get to work and had a bunch of things on my mind and forgot to do all three. While I was taking my shower, the wind blew the door shut. All I had was my towel to cover me.

My apartment was a half block from campus, so several people were always walking by. It was a sunny afternoon, so the number of people who were mulling about was even larger.

My journey to get back in my apartment was to walk down the stairs outside the complex, walk to the back porch off of the back apartment, shimmy up a decorative dowel pole leading up to the roof over the porch of the lower apartment, climb on the roof, and climb in the window of my apartment with only the towel to cover me.

To my surprise, I accomplished all this without anyone so much as observing any of my actions, but the sheer thought patterns that went through my mind during the process was nerve-racking. The experience was something to be laughed at subsequently, but at the time, not so funny.

I had an interview in Detroit the Thursday after Memorial Day for a supervisory position at a food commons at a university there. I asked my girlfriend to go with me. The Tuesday night prior to this, I said something or some things that ticked her off, I guess. I do not remember what they were, but when I left that night, I did not realize that what I said had cut so deep. The next night, my girlfriend knocked on my door and said she would not be going with me, and as far as she was concerned, she never wanted to see me again. She slammed the door shut on my apartment and left.

I got up early the next morning to attend my interview. As I recall, I did not lose much sleep over the breakup but I was nervous about the interview. I figured another love lost for whatever reason. I continued my apprehensive thoughts on the way to the interview because the end of the line for my education in the food service supervision program was closing in, and I still did not have a job or rumors of a job.

After the interview, I was not real sure how it went I felt good about some parts and disappointed in other parts. I mulled it over in my mind for some time as I left Detroit. Then, for some reason, I wanted to share my thoughts with someone. I thought, I wish I could talk to the lady who was my girlfriend before the Tuesday uprising; she was always a good listener. Once I got back to my college town, I headed straight to her house. I draw a blank on what words I used to get back in her life, but whatever I said worked. I am sure they were in order of apology. I think she had cooled off a little also, so my petitions were accepted.

I proceeded to share my discomfort with the interview. She encouraged me with positive words in my behalf. A year or two later, I looked back on this forty-eight-hour-plus engagement as the one incident that was a turning point in my future commitment to one person.

On June 20, 1969, after my present girlfriend and I visited her sister in the hospital (she had given birth to a son), I asked my girlfriend to marry me on the way home. She accepted. I believe that day I came to her with the olive branch was the moment when we both discovered how much we cared for each other and needed each other.

One night sometime between "the incident" and my request for her hand in marriage, I discovered a link between my past and my wife-to-be.

When I was dating the resident assistant, one day we decided to get an ice cream cone at an establishment near campus. There was a cute girl working there that I had seen several times when visiting the location; I thought she was the owner's daughter.

We purchased two cones. It was rather windy that day, and when we walked outside, my lady took a few steps and the ice cream blew off her cone. We returned to the counter to explain our plight. The one girl working said she would give us another cone, but the cute girl said no, that this had been a ploy by others to get different cones when they did not like the flavor. After some discussion, I realized I was getting nowhere and left, but before I left, I told the cute girl that I would not ever return to the business.

The shop was attached to a bowling alley and a pizza establishment. The night of discovery, the subject came up because my girlfriend wanted to take her mother bowling, and I told her of the incident and I had misgivings against patronizing the business which was owned by the same person. My girlfriend proceeded to tell me she was probably that cute gir,l because she worked there at that time.

She also informed me that a friend of her old boyfriend's had experienced a similar occurrence, and she did not give him a break either, because he was a bit of a jerk and indeed tried to pull the ruse. I discovered this dude was the old boyfriend of my old girlfriend from Southeastern college. A "small world" of connections of boyfriends and girlfriends.

I had an interesting interview with a motel/restaurant in the city south of my college town for a management position. The interviewer had me do a timed test on putting wood widgets that were squares, triangles, circles, and rectangles in like holes as fast as I could a test you might have in kindergarten. The interviewer, after the interview was complete, told me he thought I had all the tools of management and the tools of food service operations, but I did not put the widgets in fast enough, so I might as well forget a hire. I guess I was a square peg in a round hole for that job, or I was not a "hole" person.

A few days before my marriage proposal, I found a position with a restaurant chain which had several burger joints around Detroit as a trainee to be a district manager over a number of the units within a certain area. The man who hired me was a graduate of the program at my college and had achieved a great deal in a short time.

I started working June 24, 1969. My friend from the apartment house had found a job working for a health department in the Detroit area for the summer, and we shared an apartment.

The job was going rather well until after five weeks, Uncle Sam sent greetings he wanted my services. My fiancée' and I had planned on getting married in November 1969. When the drafting came to the front, further discussion commenced.

I had a medical problem that existed as a result of a hairline fracture of my skull near my right ear when I was in the car accident in which my mother was killed. I was told by the doctor whose care I was under, after the accident, to obtain a recommendation from an ear, nose, and throat specialist if I was ever called in the service.

I wrote a letter to the director of the local draft board to ask for an extension to allow me to visit a doctor. My fiancée asked me to marry her sooner if I got this extension. The extension was granted, and we were married August 30, 1969.

My future wife and I had to take abridged prenuptial counseling sessions required by our church. At this time, the girl I had dated who wished to get a degree in spousal science was also taking instructions. One day she and her future husband were coming in for one of their meetings, and we had just completed one of our sessions and were leaving. She acted like she did not know me. I saw her and her husband years later in church; they had eight children.

I had obtained the medical opinion and took it with me when I left for the induction physical with several other gentlemen on September 6, 1969. One out of every five men were drafted into the Marines. I was lucky enough to be chosen as one of these future Marines as part of preliminary actions I had taken.

I responded incorrectly to a question from the gentleman who was our first contact in the process, and I received a reactionary five-minute chewing out regarding proper methods of addressing any requests for feedback and any request made by those in authority. I in turn indicated that I fully understood my error. Another gentleman who was my peer, commented that the man in charge could go have relations with himself, who did he think he was, and that this was the only job he probably ever had in the man's army. This was not met well, to say the least, and I never saw this fellow again in the remaining time I spent at this site. I was sent home due to my medical condition.

One of the fellows who left with me that day was injured in Vietnam to a point that he was to be confined to a wheelchair the rest of his life. Another man was killed in the war. I never saw either of them again.

When I returned on the bus that had taken us there, my best man in my wedding gave me a ride back to our apartment in my college town.

My wife and I decided that Detroit was not the place for us to live, as we were more small-town people. She was working at a supermarket as a cashier; I worked odd jobs and for a pizza place doing a variety of jobs there. I was interviewing for jobs in the meantime.

In late October, my wife informed me the time of the month had not happened.

In mid-November, I obtained a job as a manager trainee for a fast food establishment near the city south of my college town. I was placed at this location where I would be trained to take over a location in another city near Lake Michigan. The manager who was to train me resented me, because he had worked for the company for fourteen years prior to being promoted to the manager position. He flat-out told me that being a "college boy," I should not be able to step into the position our boss had indicated I was being trained for. He also had a young man working for him as assistant manager who had worked for him since he was sixteen years old and was now nineteen years old, who he thought should get the position.

These two fellows did not cut me any slack and tried to ambush me from the promotion. The manager told me several times he thought I had the book knowledge to a point, but I did not have the total package of mechanical skills and mental skills that were needed to work in a restaurant, let alone try to manage one.

To add insult to injury the nineteen year old young man would work his tail off when his manager or the owner were around but loafed when they were not present. Many times he would sit out in the dining room and talk for long periods of time with his friends or sit in the office with his feet up and take a nap. Some of our employees told me I should report him. After we worked a shift together, he would report to the people above us that I had not performed this or that duty exactly right, in his opinion. I put up with this until one night my wife came in to tell me the results of her doctor appointment as per her carrying our child. I sat with her for a few minutes, and she left and I went back to work.

The next day when I came in to work, the manager wanted to talk to me. He said, Golden Boy had told him I sat with my wife for an hour talking during a busy time. I rebutted that this was not true; however, he should talk. This started a who-is-lying-to-who battle. The employees were afraid to take sides, and the manager told me he never saw Golden Boy loaf or experienced him lying before. So the war was on.

I decided after a few months that this life was not for me.

# TALE TWENTY-FOUR

## For the Ħealth of Ħt

ONE DAY A REPRESENTATIVE OF the health department came in. This perked my interest and brushed off the small line of cobwebs that had gathered since leaving school. About the same time, I learned of an opening at the same health agency that performed the inspection of our establishment.

I had to take a test first. I took the test and scored well, but my lack of a degree in a science-related field disqualified me. Each day at the food service unit became less encouraging. I discussed returning to college with my wife some.

We rented an upstairs apartment. Three rooms had been converted into a bedroom, a kitchen/sitting room/dining area, and a living room, with a tiny bathroom with a stool and sink off the living room. The remaining portion of the upper level of the house was a bedroom for the owner's son. The man and woman who owned the house lived in the lower level. We had to go downstairs to the back utility room to take a shower. This proved interesting during the winter. You did not linger long after taking the shower in the winter, as the only access to the apartment was an outside stairs. The owners could also monitor our bathing practices.

The couple and their son were really nice people. We became close in a short period of time. I discussed my thoughts regarding returning to school with them. The gentleman said, "You can never go wrong with more education." Three of their children had four-year degrees, and their son who was still at home was in his first year of college. The rent money from the apartment had been providing money for their offspring's education.

After a little more discussion with my wife, it was agreed that I would go back to school after the baby was born, and my wife would return to her job at the supermarket in my college town.

During the last three weeks of employment with the food chain, I spent time with another manager at another location. After a week of working with me, he thought I was more than capable to work in the food industry. He tried to get me to stay with the company. He said he would put in a good word for me with the owners. He said I could continue training with him, and I could go far in the organization. He almost convinced me to stay; however, I had already enrolled in college, and my plans were made.

The third week in May of 1970, I hit the road and did not look back anymore at any thoughts of remaining with the restaurant corporation. I was still a bit apprehensive about the math and chemistry, but I planned only to obtain an associates degree, so I would only need to take one chemistry class and one math class.

My wife was due to have our child the last week in May or the first week in June. She was going to go back to work at the supermarket the first week in July. That was her plan, anyway.

My first day of classes was to be June 4, 1970. I had a chemistry class right off the bat and a law class. No classes were offered in the summer in my major. I had obtained a job making wooden boxes to transport parts, small and large, which were manufactured at other factories including General Motors. The job's work hours were from 4:00 p.m. to 1:00 a.m. My plan was to attend classes in the morning and work the designated hours.

The job at the box factory did not require a great deal of education. Just bring your own hammer and learn how operate a nail gun. The foreman interpreted the blueprint and showed the workers how to construct the units according to the specifications.

My wife had our baby on June 8, 1970. Three things occurred which put my further education on hold.

First: The first day I reported to work I was told to come back the next day, as I was going to be working from 7a.m. to 4 p.m.

Second: My wife could not go to work until the first week in August, doctor's orders.

Third: I called in sick two days, June 4 and June 6th. to attend chemistry class I needed to decide whether to stay with the job or attend class. The class was worse than I imagined. I thought Sister was right ("Gerry, do not take math or science classes"). I dropped both classes and put all my effort into working..

The working conditions were not the best; it was hotter than blazes in the shop most days. The mechanical equipment left something to be desired.

One day early in July, I was operating a nail gun, and I was attempting to join two pieces of wood on an angle. The gun ejected one nail after I pulled the trigger, but another followed, taking a different route and piercing the area of my hand between the pointer finger and the thumb. I pulled the three-inch nail out of my left hand with my right hand. The nail had found its way through my hand to almost the head portion. Since I had a nail on my four fingers and one thumb, I did not feel I needed an extra one.

I went to the office where our secretary, a man who had a great deal of feminine qualities, was sitting speaking on the phone. He said, "Just a minute; I will be with you after this phone call. I waited a minute then I showed him my wound. He then hung up the phone and yelled, "Oooh! Oooh! Oooh! We must take you for medical assistance!"

In those days, doctors were more readily available in their office for emergency situations. I went to my wife's baby doctor (He was an adult doctor not a doctor who was a baby.) He worked on the area and flushed the area of the wound out. No stitches were needed, as basically it was a puncture wound. The doctor placed a gauze bandage on the area and said I was good to go. He gave the standard, "If you have any problems, check back with me or the hospital.

My wife had just left the office fifteen minutes before my arrival after a follow-up visit for her and the baby. She had dropped me off at work, so she had the Biscayne.

The doctor asked if I wanted any pain medication. I, being one who enjoyed at times bragging about how I could endure pain, declined. The secretary asked me if I wanted to go home for the remaining portion of the day. I told him I needed the money and continued work would not bother me, and that my wife would be coming to pick me up, so I would not need to drive myself home.

The remaining portion of the day went well, and I was able to do my work. When my wife arrived to pick me up, I received a goodly amount of sympathy from her. Pain was not a problem until the moment I went to bed. It felt like every time my heart beat, a nail was going through my hand again. About 4:00 a.m., I fell asleep from exhaustion. I went to work the next day; work took my mind off the pain. The next night was not as bad, and as time went on the pain subsided and I healed. I did not let on to anyone about the pain besides my wife.

About three or four days later, a coworker approached me about becoming a member of a gang he was forming. (When we were at lunch a couple of days after he arrived on the scene, he mentioned to some of us that he had just got out of jail for some sort of stealing.) His reason for wishing me to be a member of his gang was because I showed so much toughness with the nail gun incident

I, of course, declined his offer. I thanked him for his consideration, as I had only been asked a couple times before to be a member of an organized group, the Boy Scouts and a fraternity. My dad said he could not afford the Boy Scouts for me, and the same pretty much ran true for me personally regarding the fraternity. He was pleasant about my refusal and said, " I just thought I would ask."

About a month later, he was arrested for stabbing someone in a bar.

My wife went back to work the first week in August. I enrolled in college again to take sixteen credit hours after discussion with my best man, my friend who was still in the environmental health program, and my wife. They all encouraged me, saying they thought I could make it through the science and math.

A short time before I was to return to school, the foreman informed the company he was leaving. I was approached about filling the position. I had learned to read the prints for patterns for building the products we constructed, and had been assisting the foreman in setting up the projects for some time.

Some of the workers would take restroom breaks several times a day during the first few weeks I worked at the shop. The "breaks" were basically for smoking purposes. The foreman had to check on these characters frequently to tell them to get back to work. I told them a few times that if they did not start listening to the foreman, they could get fired. The standard comeback when someone was presented with the option of being fired was, "I was looking for a job when I came here." This general work ethic throughout the shop was the attitude of many of the individuals causing a substantial turnover rate.

Goosing each other with the handle of a hammer was commonplace.

Other characters who had been working at the factory for some time would head to the bar after we were paid on Friday and drink most of the night. Some also had families.

After I had worked at the shop for a while, I would discuss my plans for the future with some of the fellows during legal breaks and lunch. Some of them questioned my work ethic, since I would not be working for long at my present source of employment. I basically told them, a day's work for a day's pay. Some men seemed to change their attitude, started not "smoking in the boys' room" and putting a little more effort into the tasks at hand. I was surprised that I did not get some comments about butt kissing; maybe they did this behind my back.

The powers that be, including the secretary and exiting foreman, felt my example-setting showed good management skills and my ability to catch on quickly to our general daily work routine were good reasons for me to be offered the position of foreman. The workers thought I should take the advancement also; they said they would work for me. I had thoughts of accepting the position, but because of the encouragement of my wife and friends that I could make the grade in the program I had enrolled in, I chose to turn down the offer.

I did not mention the offer to my wife right off. I was sort of on an emotional seesaw regarding my potential, for becoming successful in some occupation. Some individuals had given me good opinions regarding my potential, and others had not. I questioned myself whether my future may be cast in a job like working in a factory as foreman or supervisor.

We purchased our mobile home in mid-August after renting a so-called basement house our first couple months back to my college town. A bird flying in through the fireplace on two occasions pushed forward my wife's thoughts of purchasing a mobile living unit.

With payments on this unit and basic necessities for the two of us and our daughter, for fall and winter terms, the money was fixed. Besides my wife working, I worked for my manager friend and worked cleaning buildings during the fall and winter break. I did not work a great deal for my manager friend, because I took sixteen credit hours during fall term and twenty-one credits winter during term.

I remember taking our daughter out for a ride in the snow using a cardboard box with a piece of twine for a sled that winter. We did not have much money for entertainment, but those were wonderful times together with our daughter. We had the dachshund too for a little while, but we both had mixed feelings about him.

To my surprise, chemistry class was not that bad after all, although the teacher was a jerk. He scheduled a test for the opening day of deer hunting, November 15, after several of the students asked him to schedule it another day. He had a proctor give the test and went hunting himself with his sons. He bragged the next time we had a class about their successful hunt.

I did not set the world on fire, but did okay. During the winter term in my algebra class, I was the guy who kept the grade curve high, as I had the highest grade in the class. This accomplishment was the first and last time I ever obtained this status.

I spent the spring of 1971 actually working for a local health department as part of a required co-op program for my major. I received sixteen credit hours for this training. For most students at other locations throughout the state, it was following the workers around each day learning the profession and putting together a special project. For me after two weeks of training, I actually worked in the field and office performing services such as restaurant inspections. I fit in well and discovered pretty much this occupation was going to be for me.

I will always remember the first complaint I was asked to handle. The complaint was sewage on the ground at a residence out in the rural area. My boss/trainer drove to the location and sent me to the door to discuss the issue with someone at the site. It was a Friday afternoon, and I had mixed emotions, hoping somewhat that no one would be home so I could think about the situation a bit more, and on the other hand, wanting to get my feet wet for the first time. Nobody was home; I breathed a sigh of relief.

The following Monday, I was sent out on my own to visit the site. On the way I was rather nervous. This time somebody was home, and I handled the situation.

After that I hit the ground running. I was well liked by the staff and was hired for the summer to work as a staff person. I, of course, did not get paid for my co-op, but I was paid an acceptable wage for the summer staff position.

At the end of the term, I was required to put on at least an hour-and-a-half-to-two-hour presentation. I was worried I did not have enough material for the presentation and realized I was not the greatest speaker in the world. Once I got started, I had more than enough information as I recalled many of my experiences along with other parts of the topics, which were required to be touched upon.

I received an A on my time spent at the local health department, and the same for my presentation.

The summer work went just as well as the co-op.

One day I visited a site where a house existed. The people who lived there had a son who was getting married, and he wished to place a mobile home not too far from the existing residence. These people were really nice, and they had a down-home attitude about them. They let their chickens be anywhere they pleased, and a hog sort of had the run of the place. I was required to do one or more borings to check the soil and water table conditions on the property.

While I was performing the boring, one the chickens came up and pooped on my shoe. The mother said to the chicken, "You had ant done that to the man's shoe." The father and mother first chased the chicken away, then the mother grabbed a towel off the washline and wiped my shoe off. I had lifted my foot up on a tree stump for her to wipe it off, and as I was doing this, another chicken ran up and pooped on the other shoe. The father said, "You probably think we train the chickens to do that to government workers, don't you." I just smiled. He furthermore said, " I knows who is going make right nice eaten' for dinner for us tonight." The hog started heading in my direction. The mother said, "Do not worry about her; she will not poop on you. She is shy around strangers."

After the summer was over, a position opened at the health department. All those who had worked with me tried to talk me into taking the position. I had one more class to take towards my two-year degree and I had made up my mind to obtain a bachelor's degree in my program. If I took the job, I probably could have taken the class and also worked, but to get the other degree would have been a slow process, and many of the program classes were during the work hours. So I chose to complete the program for my bachelor's degree and have a little less money.

Half of the classes I took in the fall 1971 and during winter and spring terms of 1972 were in my major; the other half were three chemistry classes, a microbiology class, a trigonometry class, a zoology class, a physics class, a drafting class, a law class, and an entomology class. Again, I did not set the world on fire in these classes, but I made average-to-a-little-above-average grades.

I had some problems with the physic class. I had some debates with the instructor about gaining credit for my answers. He was a stickler about having every detail of an answer to a problem. You could have the correct answer, but if you left a word or number out by accident on your way to the answer of a problem, he would not allow credit for any portion of the answer. Other students also contended he could be more liberal with his judgment of our answers and also made a plea for their cases. We would have ten 10-point problems. Having one or two of these questions not accepted could reduce your over-all score quickly.

One day and night just before Thanksgiving 1971, we had a bad snowstorm. Our class was from 5:00 p.m. to 6:15 p.m. When we got out of class, there was understandably a great deal of snow. My car was parked along the street, two cars behind our professor's. I noticed that he was not going to get out of his parking space without some help, as he was, in essence, stuck in the snow. I had a shovel in my car, and after a short time I had him on his way. I did not have any trouble getting out, as the Biscayne did not let me down, and the area where I was parked was not as drifted.

I had two tests and three laboratory sessions after that. The professor without a doubt was charitable with his review of my efforts; credit was given more freely after the snow episode. I believe similar pains were taken in my regard on the final exam, as I ended up with a respectable grade after starting out with a below-average grade level the first weeks of the term.

I was having a little trouble with my last chemistry class, so I obtained a student tutor the fourth week of the spring term. The young lady the college service set me up was a very attractive lady. By the third week of our two meetings per week, I had advanced to the point that I was no longer having problems; however, I found it pleasant to meet with her. I attempted to act like I was not fully understanding the material. My acting must have not been worthy of an Oscar, because the fourth week she said to me, "Mr. Martin, I believe you do not need my help any longer, and other students are more in need of my services." A combination of my poor acting and the young lady checking with the instructor regarding my status in the class ended my run with her. I had no thoughts of any relationship, plus I always discussed my wife and daughter with her. I just enjoyed the atmosphere. I told my wife of my ploy when the meetings ended. She said I was a goofball.

Our zoology instructor had what he called a pop quiz, which did not have much of a pop to it. He had a quiz before each class. The quizzes consisted of ten fill-in-the-blank questions he would put on an overhead. There were three characters who I guess were not always prepared for the quiz. They'd sit behind other students in the theater-style classroom and copy off them. One day they sat behind me and started copying off my paper. I turned around and said to them, " I am barely passing this course, so I would not copy off me." One of them said, " Sure you are." I had been doing pretty well in the class; however, on this quiz I did not do so well. We would get the quizzes back at the beginning of the next class. The three birds moved to another area when we received this particular quiz results.

This same instructor, the first day of our class, had us fill in the standard answer sheet A,B,C,D randomly without any questions. We did not know the purpose until the next class. The instructor took a test that he had given previously and used it as a guideline to compare what we would have scored on the test by just guessing at the answers. A little over half of the class would have received a passing grade as per the final outcome of his experiment.

I have always had trouble taking timed test; give me a test with no restrictions and I always do rather well. I took my trigonometry class in the winter of 1972. The instructor was a crooked, decaying-toothed man whose hygiene practices left something to be desired. He waltzed through problems as fast as he could and cut sessions short and did not entertain very many questions. He said you either get this stuff or you don't. When he saw someone struggling, he would get a big old grin on his face and show those crooked, decaying teeth.

I did get the "stuff," in fact, I tutored my best friend in the program during this go-around in my education. We would go to the library, and I helped him with problems he had troubles with. Many times he was lost, and I got him back on track.

When I took a test in the trigonometry class, I froze because the instructor gave us twenty to twenty-five problems to complete and would give us until ten minutes before the session was over. If you have ever solved a trigonometry problem, you know you must label sine, cosine, tangent, and cotangent functions properly. So providing the information correctly for Mr. Unsanitary was very tedious.

My buddy aced, the first three tests, and I got a high C. The fourth test I aced and so did my buddy, because I had learned not to be so uptight. My buddy and I sat next to each other each class. "Old Tooth Decay" accused me of cheating off my friend's paper. He gave me that trademark smile when he told me. My buddy explained to him how I had helped him. I tried to explain to him that it would be awfully difficult to copy all the data for every problem, as complicated as it was to write down the information to begin with. He would not give in right away, but after bit more discussion, he said he would give me twenty more similar problems and would make arrangements to have someone proctor the test at a special time. This test went well, I got an even better score, plus the proctor did not rush me. The instructor was cordial to me the rest of the term, and I received a decent grade.

The spring term of 1972, I took twenty-four credit hours of classes to cut down on my time spent. Two-thirds of the classes were only offered during the spring term. Taking them at that time meant I could graduate winter term of 1973. One of the classes in my major was a slam dunk for me, because it was sort of an extension of a class I took in the food program; it was a communicable disease class. A drafting class was a similar slam dunk, because it involved using the same skills I had learned from working at the "box" factory and from a couple classes in the food program.

The woman who taught the drafting class, or should I say made her presence known, was for the most part putting her time in prior to retirement. The class was held once a week for an hour and half from 4:30 p.m. to 6:00 p.m. The teacher would take attendance, then lecture for fifteen or twenty minutes, and then we would work on a design project that coincided with our choice field. The project was like a term paper, more or less. We did not have any tests. The project was our grade for the term.

The teacher sometimes could not put two sentences together that made sense. By fall term 1972, she had been encouraged to retire.

One day she told us when she was having a good day that she had obtained a degree in engineering, but she was basically blackballed from positions because she was a woman. My college offered her a position to teach in the Technical and Industrial Arts program, so she took it. She said she liked being around students. I was told that at one time she was a very bright, highly regarded, and knowledgeable instructor. A few times she showed us this was true on her good days. I remember she once said, "When performing a task, see what is likely to happen, then give careful thought in planning your final product." She also said on another occasion, "If you are part of the solution, the problem is reduced or solved." I personally tried to follow those suggestions a number of times in my life.

I worked at the food unit for my manager friend at 5:00 p.m. each day. The drafting class was the only class that interfered with my job once per week. Since the teacher did not provide too much assistance, sometime after she started her lecture, I would leave for my job. On the days she appeared to have it together, I stayed until she was done and then left. A couple times when she took attendance, she said, "Mr. Martin, I do not remember you being in this class."

I completed my project on my own time. My project was the plans for a mobile home park similar to the park we lived in.

The last day of the class, I stayed the whole time and finished some things I purposely left for completion in the class. Our instructor looked at it and said to others in the class, "Now this is what I tried to show you-how a proper project should be put together and completed. I guided this student through this work, and now we have a excellent product." I do not know who she thought she guided through the work that term, but that was the first time she ever saw my project that entire term.

I received an A for the class. Some of my classmates were amazed that I captured the grade I did, skipping out as I did. I never knew whether I deserved it or if the instructor just had a bad day the day she completed review of the project, but I did not argue with the results.

The dean of health, science, and arts was looking for someone in the fall of 1971 to rake leaves and put up storm windows for her and some older widows. From these jobs I gathered several jobs working for other women from that time until I graduated.

My father-in-law loved to celebrate St. Patrick's Day. I am not sure how much Irish blood flowed through his veins, but he loved the Irish. He visited Ireland when he was in the army and vacationed there with my mother-in-law after he retired in 1983. He rooted for the Notre Dame Irish, although he was not fond of the Catholic faith. When something was unusual or failed to meet expectations, he said, " Don't that make you thumb your rosaries." He did not dislike Catholics; he just was not certain about the faith and said he found some Catholics to be hypocritical. I told him this could be said of every faith. I told him, "When you choose to follow a faith and try to show others your beliefs and then give in to temptation, others point fingers." He said he did not need to go to church; he had his own understanding with J.C.

My father-in-law spent many years consuming a variety of spirits on St. Patrick's Day with his friends, because to him and his friends, Irish descent was not a prerequisite for enjoying the day. I never really observed the holiday in my youth, mostly because of my German descent and the Irish differences in the area I grew up. I respected the Irish holiday more, though, when I attended high school in Southeastern Town, where the student population was largely of Irish descent. In our area, in those days, the holiday was to be celebrated only by the Irish. I never have worn green on the day, although my friends wanted me to be an honorary Irishman.

In March of 1972, St. Patrick's Day fell on Friday. My friend from the trigonometry class and my program was Irish, so he talked me into celebrating the holiday and having TGIF (Thank God it's Friday). After our last class, we headed to a bar within walking distance of campus. Both our wives had our vehicles at their work. After we had two pitchers of green beer, we decided to go to a bar about a half-mile away through town and on the north side of town. This was the first bar in the area to serve shelled peanuts where you just toss the shells on the floor.

My buddy had been a rodeo participant, riding bucking horses when he was a bit younger. He was twenty-nine years of age at the time. Five years earlier he had had an accident at a rodeo in Detroit. His sternum was cracked in three places, requiring a tracheotomy so he could have aid in breathing. He took up calf roping, which was a little more safe for him. He was still in pretty good shape, so, it being a cold evening, he talked me into running to our destination to keep warm.

After two more pitchers of green beer, we were on our way from being tipsy to an honest-to-goodness heavy buzz. My buddy really liked Jerry Lee Lewis, so he decided to play two of his songs on the jukebox. When the second song, "A Whole Lotta Shakin' Goin' On," began to play, he decided to go over to a piano nearby and emulate Mr. Lewis on the keyboard. Somewhere in the middle of the song, he chose to kick the piano bench away as Jerry Lee would do.

The piano bench action was judged-and rightly so-as improper conduct by the bartender. We were asked to depart from the premises and not return. This was the first time and still is my only time I have been barred from any establishment. Our imposed adjournment led us to go to two more bars in the middle of town, where we had another two pitchers of amber-fluid-turned-green in each house.

We then returned to the original watering hole just off campus where we had started our day of tanking up. I am not sure how many pitchers we had there, but a strobe light ended our "fun." The device caused both of us to develop a headache and an uneasiness in the stomach (it had to be the strobe, could not have been our drinking).

We decided to leave to call our wives, who we had told earlier in the day what we were up to. They decided to get together and wait until we were done celebrating. We called from a telephone booth (no cell phones those days); however, by this time in our journey, we were not clear in our minds which bar we had left. We told my friend's wife this, which caused both our wives to laugh their butts off at us. I left the phone booth and discovered a street sign about twenty-five feet from the booth. I had to ask my buddy repeatedly, "What did you say?" as I tried to relay the information as to where we were located. He was also attempting not to slur his speech to my wife, who was going to pick us up.

My wife picked us up and took my buddy home. When we arrived home, I went straight to bed, but sometime in the middle of the night I decided to try to sit on top of some textbooks, which were on top of our clothes hamper. My wife retrieved me from there, but then I decided I wanted to sleep in our bathtub. She decided to leave me there.

I awoke the next morning with a stiff neck, imagine that. My buddy called about 10:00 a.m. we both agreed that green beer did not look good in the toilet, and it was not pleasant upchucking it either.

A couple months later, my brother-in-law and I went to the bar for lunch that we had been kicked out of. I was asked to turn around the way I came in and leave the premises.

Two years later, my wife and I went to the same bar for lunch while visiting my wife's family. I wore a Chicago Cubs hat and sunglasses just in case. There were different employees, however.

The summer of 1972 was dedicated to a block of classes that combined sociality, geology, and environmental problem solving. We were guinea pigs for the program which forever thereafter was known as "The Summer Block" at the college.

Because of the blending of classes, there was also a blocking of hours of time during the day devoted to overall class time and fieldwork. Therefore, I could not work at the food commons for my friend the manager. I had mixed emotions. I lost money from not working, but on the plus side-a minor plus side-I did not need to put up with my friend's daughter bugging me about marrying a "Townie." She was now attending college and was working for her dad and managed to comment every time I saw her. She would say something like, " I was not good enough for you; I see how you are."

I was still working doing odd jobs for my group of ladies on weekends. My cowboy friend's wife worked as a secretary for the campus security office, and she found me a job directing traffic for special events. During the fall term of 1972 and winter term of 1973, I directed traffic at football games, basketball games, and music concerts that were held at the college.

The "blending of hours" occurred because we performed hands-on fieldwork such as studying rivers and natural resources. The materials and lectures overlapped each other for each class. One of the highlights of the summer block was a unexpected trip to Pennsylvania in late June and early July. The Susquehanna River had flooded over from a long period of heavy rain. The flooding influenced several areas along the river, encompassing a multiphase of miles along the river.

A highly ranked individual in Pennsylvania's environmental response division was a friend of one of our program directors, so they made an accord to have our group travel to the inundated area to aid in recovery proceedings.

We reported to the maintenance garage at the school at 6:00 A.M. to leave on our trip. The departure was delayed, however, because a safety inspection by the head of maintenance revealed an oil change was needed, and new tires were required for both vehicles. We left about 12:30 p.m.

Many of us did not get much sleep the night before. Small catnaps were taken as we rode through the night. About 1:00 a.m. the next day somewhere a few miles from Pittsburgh, the driver of our car decided to take a catnap himself while driving. The point he chose was an area where the roadside provided a considerable drop-off, and there were no guardrails. The passenger who was sitting beside him grabbed the wheel and righted the vehicle. Although the action managed to remove sedation from most everyone in the car, the incident prompted us to stop for a short time.

By this time we were pretty slaphappy. Anything one said to another became a source of laughter and silliness. One of my comrades sang to the tune of "Smoke Gets In Your Eyes" the following:

> Some people asked me why
> Raccoon feces is blue
> I simply replied
> Comes from deep inside

Everyone howled uncontrollably. (A few days later, it did not seem as funny.)

We arrived in Harrisburg, the capital about 5:30 a.m. After some discussion with the contacts we were to meet, we were taken to an armory, where we slept on some cots until about 10:00 a.m.

We then were divided up; one group was sent to Wilkes-Barre, and my group was sent to Williamsport.

An interesting observation our group had was that as we were exiting Harrisburg, although it had only stopped raining forty-eight hours prior, in a more affluent area which existed a greater elevation above the flooded area, a man was watering his grass. This was rather a paradox of concerns. The people in the flooded areas were worried about their living quarters, businesses, and possessions. The gentleman on the higher ground was worried about his blades of grass getting enough moisture.

The motel we stayed in was located uphill from the ball field for the Little League World Series at the time. The outfield fence was about five hundred yards from our windows in the motel. My cowboy buddy and I bunked together in a room.

Our job basically was to go out at 8:30 a.m. in the morning each day to monitor and estimate the amount of items that were being hauled away in dump trucks to be disposed of, in various landfills, as result of cleanup and recovery. We worked these centers until 5:00 p.m. The landfill/recovery area that we worked covered about a seventy-five mile radius.

We learned firsthand the destruction capabilities of the flooding caused by overflow of a river as the result of heavy rains. We also learned the perils that the people experience as result of the destruction.

The government's role in emergency preparedness and resource recovery was laid out for us to observe. In some cases, the Army Corps of Engineers who were in charge of operations were also learning as they went.

At night we would find different things to do. Sometimes we would drive around observing flood-damaged areas and the remnants of the damage after the water had receded. We observed how sandbags were used to try to hold back the water.

One night we decided after dinner/supper to walk to a nearby bar. I had a couple of beers with the guys and decided to return to the motel. I left a twenty-dollar bill for my two beers and told my buddy to buy a round for the boys. I told him to bring me back the change from this transaction. (eight students and two instructors were the boys). A beer was sixty cents in those days. The next morning I asked my buddy for my change. He gave me one dollar and twenty-three cents. I said, "Where is the rest?"

He said, "That is it."

I said, "What kind of deal is this?"

He said, "Next time don't leave so much money. Sometimes you learn from your mistakes."(He followed this with a snicker.)

I said, "This pisses me off."

I went to breakfast but did not say anything to anyone. After breakfast, my buddy said, "Are you still mad?"

I said, "Yes, I am."

Now my buddy had a standard response to his wife when he asked her the same question, and she responded the same as I did. It was, " If you stay mad forever, you will stay mad for a long time." This response may have contributed to his divorce a few years later. Therefore, this was his response to my "Yes, I am." I just ignored his reply.

The locations we worked at were manned by one person. A bagged lunch was provided, and you would be picked up between 4:30 p.m. and 5:00 p.m. As the day went on, I cooled off. When I was picked up, the boys who had already been picked up, including my buddy, greeted me with, "There is old money bags."

Getting my goat, I surmised, was their plan.

A priest told me when I was in high school (when I was in a situation where someone was trying to push a teasing episode) that a forest fire can be started by a small flame. He said the tongue can be the small flame, and when the two tongues battle each other, a small disagreement can turn into a war of words. When a forest fire begins to spread, it takes a lot of resources to put it out, and the forest is not the same thereafter. A war of words can leave a lifetime of emotional scars. In some cases, these words are like pouring gas on the fire. Many times in my life I have not heeded his counseling, but this time I did. I just laughed and said "Good one, guys." No further mention was made of the incident in the future.

A couple of nights later, my buddy and I walked down to the baseball field. He had salvaged a rubber ball from the landfill he worked at. We found a stick to use as a bat. We took turns pitching to each other and batting. We commented to others from that day forward that we had played baseball at the baseball diamond where the Little League World Series was held at that time. Sometimes it doesn't take much to please one.

We spent ten days total at the Williamsport and Wilkes-Barre locations. We left to go back to the college town at 7:00 a.m. We called our wives and told them we would be home between eleven and eleven thirty that night. This arrival time was based on a stop for lunch and dinner.

Somewhere around five in the afternoon we took a vote on who wanted to stop for a full-fledged dinner or who wanted to just grab a snack and be on our way. The snack idea won out. Cell phones did not exist, so we did not let anyone back home know of our change in plans.

We arrived at home near 9:00 p.m. When one of our comrades arrived home, he found his wife in bed with another man. The fellow and his wife lived behind our mobile home just one unit down. We pretty much knew this affair had been going on. When my classmate left for any extended amount of time, this gentleman arrived. Although he was in the same program and we were neighbors, we did not speak much to each other, more than a "Hi, how are you," nor did our wives. Therefore, we were not certain who the mystery gentleman was who visited the home.

The sad part about the situation was that all the time we were gone, he bragged constantly how much he and his wife loved each other and how well they got along.

A week later the mobile home had a For Sale sign in the window. I did not see him until many years later at a conference. He had married again, had two children, and was working as a consultant for a recycling company.

After our return, we spent parts of the remaining portions of the summer and portions of the fall term promoting our college through slide presentations of our trip. Our instructors and the officials of our school handled any interviews and presentations made for the most part. We were just the nonspeaking actors to be presented as symbols of the twelve-day expedition and to be paraded for publicity for the college. We had our fifteen minutes of fame as a group.

The balance of the summer block consisted of river study and study of soils of land owned by the college and by some of the instructors.

We took a ten-mile canoe trip down the largest river we studied.

When my sister was in fourth grade, two girls in her class snuck off to a gravel pit area where one of the excavated areas had been flooded with water, for the purpose of swimming. It was a Sunday afternoon. They had told each other's parents that they were going to each other's house. Therefore, it was not until about 6:00 p.m. that both parents became concerned that neither child had returned to the appropriate home. It was never discovered how they drowned.

From this tragedy, many parents in the area took the same road as my mother's family did regarding the pickles. These parents did not want their kids to take swimming lessons. The opposite, rather, should have occurred. I consequently learned to fear water and I never learned to swim.

The upshot of the trip down the river for me was that I was surrounded by lifesaving equipment. There were three of us in our canoe, with me holding on for dear life. I was not much help in rowing, especially when we went over a stretch of rapids one-half mile from our destination.

About an hour after we were in the water, we ran across an area about a quarter-mile long that had snakes hanging from trees that leaned over the water. Two fellows that were with us were alarmed and dreaded these snakes. They had teased me about my fear of water, and I teased them about their fear of snakes. One of the snakes fell in our canoe. I held it up as we went near both fellows, who were in different canoes; they both grimaced at the sight. Each of us has our own powerless moments for one reason or another. One person's fear might be another's strength or enjoyment.

We conducted a survey throughout the college town asking a number of questions regarding what the residents thought were the needs of the town and surrounding area. One question also asked what the college could do for the town. My father-in-law said, when I asked the question regarding what the college could do, "The pinheads and the college can leave town." My friend the food service manager's daughter said, "The students could marry more Townies."

That was the last time I saw his daughter. My manager friend did not let on where she went. I found out years later she left home for Oregon, where she got a job after one too many disagreements with her dad. She reconciled after an extended period of time. By this time she had obtained a degree in sociology.

During the fall term of 1972, I finally came to the realization that I could be successful in the field I had chosen to follow.

Winter term was my last term. I had two classes and understandably spent a lot of the time reviewing the job opening listings.

The term ended March 15. I had interviewed for a number of jobs in late February and early March. In late February, I interviewed with a man who was a close friend of one of our instructors/program head (and also the man who arranged our trip to Pennsylvania). The man was visiting the college to meet with a student who was to be a co-op student in the spring. He spoke with me because he was working on adding a staff member to only inspect food establishments in the county where he was the Director of the Environmental Division of the Health Department. My instructor recommended me to him.

We had a nice chat, and he gave me an application to fill out and send to him. I did not put a lot of stock in the possibility of being employed with this agency, as he indicated there were a lot of "ifs" involved with the position he was attempting to propose to his county commissioners. My instructor said it was good practice for interviewing though.

As March 15 approached, I still did not have any plausible certainty that I would be employed soon by any agency.

The second Friday of the month, I had a Interview with a local health department. My wife had to work so I asked my mother-in-law to stay by the phone at our house since I might receive a call from another local health department I had interviewed with earlier in the week. The agency was directed by a childhood friend of mine, so he said he would let me know one way or another. I completed the interview and headed back home; I felt I had performed well in the interview. I was informed that I would receive an answer either by mail or by phone.

When I entered the door of our home, my mother-in-law gave me a hug. She said, "You got the job." I was of course excited; however, I calmed down a bit when I discovered that the job was with the department of the man I had interviewed with on campus.

My mother-in-law left. About half an hour after she left, I received a call from the agency which I had interviewed with earlier in the week, informing me I had been selected for that job. I informed them of my other offer and told them I would let them know my decision on Monday.

Monday morning brought an offer for a position from the interview on Friday. I again held off on my decision. I discussed my situation with my wife and others. I finally decided to take the position with the department that I had interviewed with on campus (the food service inspection position). This did not set well with my childhood friend; he was rather cold to me when I saw him at meetings and the like. I felt bad; we had played sports together and rode the school bus together. He was there for me after my dad died. His brother bought our farm after the initial buyer sold it a few years after we left the farm. So it was not an easy decision.

My wife and I journeyed to the location of my place of employment to meet the staff, traverse the county, and find some options for placing our mobile home. The director was a great guy, confirming my choice of employment was correct. He remained so throughout the years.

When we left to return to my college town, I had several things on my mind. My first day of employment was to be April 15, 1973. I was planning in my mind the next few weeks leading up to my starting date. I took the wrong route on the expressway, which had me headed away from my proper destination. A mutual decision of my wife and I was to use an unauthorized vehicle turnaround.

As I waited for traffic to clear, one of the vehicles that approached just happened to be a State Police car. I was told to remove myself from my vehicle and get in the back of the cruiser. One the officers was pleasant, but the other was rather hard nosed (a real "grump butt" as my kids called such individuals). I was asked why I was visiting the area and a few other questions. I proceeded to ask a few questions of my own; mainly, why I was in the back of their car as result of a traffic violation? Mr. Hard Nose told me to shut up until they had finished their investigation by way of their radio.

After interchange of code numbers and police jargon, I was handed a ticket.

It still concerned me that I was sitting in the rear seat of the cruiser, when normally you were asked to stay in your vehicle on a traffic stop. I, therefore, tried again to have this concern cleared up. The pleasant officer seemed to ease off a bit (another reason for my second attempt at having an answer provided). Old "Grump Butt" however, said, "None of your business."

The officer who was more cordial proceeded to explain that they were looking for person driving a car that matched my car who had shot a fellow officer two days prior to this. He further informed me that when an officer first meets up with a person, they do not know who they are dealing with initially. I was not from the area, so hence, based on other matching concerns, they were careful when handling the situation at hand.

When the director of the division of the health department and I were discussing issues, he told me he received a very good reference from the manager of the fast food restaurant I worked at (who had admitted that he did not care much for college boys). On the way home I decided to stop and thank him for his words and thoughts in my regard.

When I walked in, Golden Boy was sitting talking to some other men (it appeared nothing had changed). I asked him if the manager was present. He said he had left to go home a half hour ago, but he was the night manager, and could he help me?

I said no and asked him if he remembered me. He said he did not. I proceeded to identify myself. He said, "Oh the college boy." I told him I went back to college and had just obtained a job at a health department. I did not indicate which one. I bid him goodbye and left him with the premise that it might be the agency who visited his establishment. I did interview with that department and used the absent manager as a reference, but a friend of mine who performed his internship there received the job.

About thirty years later, my wife and I visited a buffet restaurant with friends of ours. As we were eating, I noticed a fellow sitting in a booth during our entire visit with some men, basically just shooting the bull. I said to my friends, "He sure looks like the guy who I worked with, the Golden Boy." Prior to leaving, I went over and asked him whether he had worked at the location in question. He answered yes, but that was a long time ago. I noticed the logo of the restaurant on his shirt. He indicated that he was one of the managers.

I went back to our table. I described my work experience with the man to our friends. I said, "I must just catch him at the wrong time, finding him taking a break."

# The Lighter Side
# of the Health Environment

I STARTED WORKING AT MY NEW job on April 15, 1973, and left that environmental division on July 31, 1989.
I became employed at another health department in August of 1989 and retired from that department June 30, 2008. In my last eight years at the original department, I was the director of the division. I also took on the position of Solid Waste Coordinator for one and one-half years prior to my exit.

I began to have some health problems, so I left to take a step down to a position as a supervisor below the director of the second department. I had a lot of pressure at times, trying to be fair to the public and protect the environment. Much of the time I tried to present the intent of the laws and regulations and not the strict letter of these requirements.

Shel Silverstein wrote a composition some time in 1974 that sort of sums up my career in regards to the ups and downs of each day I perform the duties of my job.

The composition is titled "Sarah Cynthia Sylvia Stout Would Not Take The Garbage Out!"

> Sarah Cynthia Sylvia Stout
> Would not take the garbage out!
> She'd scour the pots and scrape the pans,
> Candy the yams and spice the hams,
> And though her daddy would scream and shout,
> She simply would not take the garbage out.
> And so it piled up to the ceilings:
> Coffee grounds, potato peelings,
> Brown bananas, rotten peas,

Chunks of sour cottage cheese.
It filled the can, it covered the floor,
It cracked the window and blocked the door
With bacon rinds and chicken bones,
Drippy ends of ice cream cones,
Prune pits, peach pits, orange peel
Gloppy glumps of cold oatmeal,
Pizza crusts and withered greens,
Soggy beans and tangerines,
Crusts of black burned buttered toast,
Gristly bits of beefy roasts...
The garbage rolled on down the hall,
It raised the roof, it broke the wall...
Greasy napkins, cookie crumbs,
Globs of gooey bubblegum.
Cellophane from green baloney
Rubbery blubbery macaroni,
Peanut butter caked and dry,
Curdled milk and crust of pie,
Moldy melons, dried-up mustard,
Eggshells mixed with lemon custard,
Cold French fries and rancid meat,
Yellow lumps of Cream of Wheat.
At last the garbage reached so high
That finally it touched the sky.
And all the neighbors moved away,
And none of her friends would come to play.
And finally Sarah Cynthia Sylvia Stout said,
"OK, I'll take the garbage out!"
But then, of course, it was too late...
The garbage reached across the state,
From New York to the Golden Gate.
And there, in the garbage she did hate,
Poor Sarah met an awful fate,
That I cannot right now relate
Because the hour is much too late.
But children, remember Sarah Stout
And always take the garbage out!

I will not "go there" with any of the serious parts of my thirty-five plus years of employment in the health field. But I will go there with my humorous experiences and exploits.

I already related the story of the horse buried in the barn. There are many other quirky experiences I had during those years of working at two health departments.

In my years of work, those who worked in environmental health programs throughout the state were concerned with what we were called. The names "sanitarian," "environmentalist," "environmental sanitarian," and "health inspector" were different names these professionals preferred to be called at one time or another. I really did not care what the public called us, but I did care about being called degrading names such as "that asshole." I tried to not promote those names.

Although my main purpose in my first years of employment was to inspect and oversee the requirements and procedures of restaurants and other food establishments, I also needed to learn how we handled and administered our other mandated programs that we managed. Some of these programs crossed over into the food service programs.

It was standard procedure for a new staff member to go out with each of the staff members in their assigned areas to get to know the staff member and have the new member learn the ropes in regards to their methods of dealing with the public.

There were three particular staff members with whom I spent time. One such staff member was a man who performed most of the food inspections prior to my arrival on the scene. This character was a Type A individual, on the go all the time. He owned a Volkswagen and had a lead foot.

In his area there were a few subdivisions which overlooked Lake Michigan. These developments had driving paths that elevated, were winding, and had deeper drop-offs as you proceeded to advance up the paths. There were spots where you could meet a car, but the paths were basically dirt two tracks. It seemed like every day I went out with this mentor, we had one request to visit one of these developments to check out properties to observe whether they would meet requirements in regards to codes. Each time he would speed up the paths, taking curves with hellbent fury, and do the same on the way back down the path.

On about the fourth trip, I said something to him about the roller coaster ride. He laughed and said, "Oh, I have everything under control. I never killed anyone yet, but I will slow down so you will not need to check your drawers. I'd hate to see you quit because of me; that would mean that I would need to do food establishments again, and I am not interested in doing the majority of them again." After that, the ride was a little less exciting, or else I got more accustomed to his driving.

I said something concerning the man's driving to another "sanitarian" about six months after I started employment. He said, "Yea, he does tend to have a lead foot and make any journey a bit exciting." I worked with him about three years, but I don't recall him ever getting a ticket, or at least he never let on that he did.

One day about a month after my employment, I was asked to follow up on a complaint regarding liquid waste on the surface of the ground at a residence.

When I approached the residence, I noticed the door of the tattered home was ajar. When I rapped on the door, a large hog came moseying out to greet me. No one but this hog came to the door, so I knocked again a second time. The hog only grunted, so the conversation between the hog and I was limited.

Finally, after the third knock, someone answered my request for dialogue. A heavyset women said to the hog, "Why Sonny, you should have came and got me and told me someone was here." I discussed with the lady my reason for visiting her home. A few minutes later, another hog joined Sonny, the lady, and me. As I remember, I think her name was Florence.

We proceeded to travel to the location of the final disposal of waste from the home. Indeed, there was a problem. Sonny and Florence, however, who had followed us to the site, seemed to shy away from the pollution.

A number of years later, I received a call that two sons of a lady were dipping sewage out of a septic tank with a pail and throwing the waste at each other.

I found this hard to believe. I visited the site. The mother of the two boys said when I questioned her regarding the complaint, "Oh, we have been having troubles with our system, and I told the two of them to just dip it out of the tank and dump it back in the woods, but they get going and start throwing it at each other." I informed her of the consequences of having a system that was not working and the health-related concerns. After I left her, as I was driving down the road, I thought again about the hogs years earlier, and how they shied away from the sewage. Now two human boys were playing in it.

Diphtheria, anyone?

There were many new codes and laws that were implemented in the state of Michigan from 1966 to 1969. Many of the requirements of the 1969 Food Code were covered in city and other municipality ordinances prior to its adoption, but in rural areas the rules were not too specific. Many rural area food services prior to 1969 were inspected mostly on a complaint basis. As a result, the new codes and laws for health department staffs were beefed up (no pun intended).

When I came on the scene at this generally rural agency, many food establishments had not been inspected frequently (the reason for my existence at this department). My first visit to many establishments, therefore, was to introduce myself and discuss the new requirements of the code, to make certain they understood what was expected. My inspections were mostly cursory.

After three months on the job, I had visited at least half of the licensed facilities. At this time, I also started working on mobile units that traveled from place to place serving food. We did not have a large number of these units at that time.

There was a man whose home base I had difficulty finding. I asked one of the sanitarians how I could get in touch with him. He said he lived with a farmer and his wife and that I could call him at a number that was in the establishment file.

I shared an office with the racecar driver. All of a sudden, he and my boss who had the office next to our office left abruptly for parts unknown when I began dialing the number. A man who was evidently the farmer answered the phone. I asked for the unit operator. He said, "Just a minute." There was a substantial wait, and then the man came to the phone. The man stuttered and was difficult to understand. A muddled conversation ensued between the man and me.

There was a swinging door to the office of the gentleman who gave me the phone number. As I looked to my left and tried to continue my conversation, I saw my boss, the racer, and the culprit who gave me the phone number peeking through the door, laughing their butts off.

After I hung up it was explained to me that along with the stuttering problem, he was a bit mentally handicapped, and that you needed to speak to him in person. I was told, further, exactly where his home base was. I spent many years with this gentleman operating his concession. Even when I became director of the department, I continued to handle his licensure. It was difficult sometimes getting through to him because of his disabilities, but he was a hardworking man. He also worked for the area fruit growers when he was not peddling his food wares. I had to pleasantly tell him to clean himself up sometimes when he was operating his unit. I never really knew his age until 1979. He always looked about seventy-years-old-plus from the first time I set eyes on him. When he came in our office that day in 1979, he told me had just turned sixty-eight years of age. I told him he did not look that old.

The fellow who had played the phone trick on me, overheard me tell him this. When the gentleman left, he came into my office and said, "I don't believe you," and shook his head.

When I first began to visit them, a number of food establishments were using home canned jams and jellies for breakfast service. Only freezer jams and jellies were allowed, other than commercially processed ones. I stopped in at a particular restaurant one day for an early lunch; I was sitting away from the center of the dining area, in a corner.

A customer came in. After some discussion with the waitress, she asked her why they no longer provided the jams that had previously been available. The waitress said, "Oh, some a---hole from the health department came in and told us we could not serve them anymore." The owner overheard this and called the waitress over, and I saw her point toward me. The waitress quickly placed her hand over mouth and became wide-eyed. The owner came over and apologized. I said, "That's okay, I find it particularly humorous."

From April 1973 to May 1974, I reported to a building that existed ten miles east of our residence. In this small building, our division conducted business; other divisions within our department did their business in two other venues close by in the same municipality. In May 1974, all divisions united and moved to a building constructed for our department and the Department of Social Services, three and a half miles west of our residence.

Staff meetings became part of my employment the first week in 1973. In my thirty-five-plus years of work in the health field, I was a participant in a plethora of meetings, many as a general participant, and many as the person who conducted the meetings as an administrator. The meetings in the small buildings were conducted in a space area in the racer's office and mine. The staff would huddle around a small portable table sitting in our mobile office chairs (confined-space requirements were not in effect yet). The new building possessed a very comfortable, user-friendly conference room.

I can't remember a time I attended a meeting that coffee was not available for consumption. Many times an assortment of baked goods were made available in my early years, but not so much in later years at my first location of employment and the second location. Healthy eating became more important, and fruits or vegetables were more apparent when something extra was provided.

The third member of our staff who shared the same position as me in those early days, had very deep pockets when it came to sharing with others. A number of times during the first two months of my employment, he asked me to go to lunch with him at an Oriental food establishment near our office. Each time he was "a little short" on money when it came time to pay the bill. He would ask me to cover a certain portion of his bill that he lacked.

He never volunteered to pay me back at any time. Finally after the fifth or sixth, time I approached him regarding the money he owed me. He said, " I was going to talk about that very thing today. We will go to lunch today, and I will pay for yours." Although the projected amount would not cover the amount he owed me, I agreed, because I felt at least I would recover part of his debt to me. When it came time to pay, he said, "Oh, I was going to write a check but forgot I wrote a check for my truck repair, and see, I would overdraw my account if I wrote a check for both our meals, but payday is at the end of the week, and if you pay for your meal, I will catch you Monday." Payday came and left, and there was no mention of paying me.

The following week I asked Deep Pockets to go out to lunch together at his favorite location. I ordered one of the higher-priced items on the menu, plus I ordered a meal to go. I told the waitress to keep an eye out when I was half done with my meal and put the order in for the meal to go. Deep Pockets always went to the restroom to brush his teeth after he finished his meal. When he headed for the restroom, I left my tip, headed for the door with the to-go order, and I told the waitress my companion would pay the bill. The mobile unit jester was in the parking lot to give me a ride. I gave him the to-go order for his efforts, although he was not a fan of Chinese food.

The incident was never discussed further by Deep Pockets.

When baked goods were purchased, Deep Pockets would eat his share, but he would never purchase any items for any meeting. Soon it became fashionable to buy four items unless we had a guest. When a guests were present, we made sure more items were available. Deep Pockets would always eat his share; guilt never seemed to cause him discomfort.

It has been said that no man is an island. Deep Pockets was pretty much an island. Most of the time when we discussed an issue, he was on the opposite side of the issue. Four against one was the norm.

In 1976, Racer Car Driver left to obtain a master's degree in public health administration. The four and one discrepancy remained intact with his replacement.

On one occasion, about three months had elapsed between staff meetings. An issue had been discussed at a previous meeting. The two other general staff members and I decided to find out what would happen if we took the position Deep Pockets had taken at that meeting. True to his contentious attitude toward the group, he took the position the three of us had taken at the previous meeting.

Much of the time, our boss did not see eye to eye with him. Our boss was a very calm, gentle person who was slow to anger. One day, however, he and Deep Pockets had a discussion in which Deep Pockets would not agree to take our director's recommendation. Our boss became so upset that he told Deep Pockets to go in a darkroom and wait for his brain to develop. Later in the day, he apologized to the staff and Deep Pockets for the "brain development" comment.

One day Deep Pockets brought a thirty-inch sapling into the office, in a large pot. His purpose was to study its growth. After it had reached a height of about four feet we poured several types of liquids in the pot. Coffee, orange juice, apple juice, all types of soda, and milk were examples of the liquids that were poured in the container.

The tree continued to grow at a very rapid rate. Deep Pockets commented several times that the nutrients he added to the pot must have made the tree grow so rapidly. He recorded his conclusions on a writing pad.

It was this type of functioning at work that caused our boss to be at odds with Deep Pockets. Our boss felt he spent too much time studying elements that did not have much to do with our job description.

One day when the tree had reached about six inches from the eight-foot ceiling in Deep Pocket's office, our boss told him to remove the tree from the premises. This was met with a great deal of opposition from the mortmain of the tree. A memo was necessitated before the tree was removed. My comrades and I placed our hats near our hearts in my office as Deep

Pockets wrestled the pot and the tree out the door. Several individuals, including all of us and the custodial staff, offered to assist him, but he insisted on playing the martyr.

On another occasion, Deep Pockets kept bragging for an extended amount of time about the gas mileage he was getting with his pickup. He recorded the statistics on a clipboard which he left hanging on a hook. He spent about an hour, the day he started keeping a record, attaching the hook to the wall outside his cubicle.

The recording became a steady, everyday occurrence.

We decided to pool our money to purchase three gallons of gasoline. One of us, on our break, would add this fuel to his gas tank once per week for a month. He commented that a tune-up he just had performed might be the result of his now even better mileage results.

We waited two weeks after we stopped adding the gasoline, then we siphoned about one gallon of fuel out of the tank each week for two weeks. He continued to record the information about a month after we stopped the siphoning. Then one day the clipboard was removed. We never knew whether he discovered what we had been doing or what.

I mentioned coffee was always a must at staff meetings. "Race Car" always wanted his share of coffee. He complained several times that when someone poured him a cup, they did not fill the cup full enough..

One time we took a break from our meeting, while Race Car was out of the room. I filled his cup to the brim, to a point that he could not lift the cup; he had to lean down to the cup to sip it. When he came back, he said, "Now there's a cup of coffee." Even Deep Pockets thought it was funny.

Coffee, however, became a liability at one event. This particular meeting was held when I was director of my division. We had a special administrative staff meeting. These meetings were conducted by our medical director.

A guest from our advisory board was present. A controversial issue was being discussed. Our dentist and the guest had a serious difference of opinion. As the discussion continued, it became really heated. One thing led to another, and the advisory person threw his cup of coffee at the dentist. The coffee did not reach any part of the dentist's person, but a good share of it landed on a number of official documents which were recorded in our files. The stains remained as a reminder of that fateful meeting each time someone retrieved one of the files. In fact, new staff members would ask me what the deal was when they happened to run across one of these files. This probably continued after I left the department, but possibly no explanation was forthcoming after those who were present at the meeting were longer employed at the agency.

A few days after the incident, our medical director, who had a very dry sense of humor and had spent several years in the armed forces, remarked he had seen many weapons, but that it was the first time he saw coffee used as a weapon. He said, "Maybe we needed to prohibit coffee from meetings in the future, or have each person attending a meeting carry a protective device."

Spray 'n Wash and coffee stains have become part-time friends on my shirts throughout the years. Turbulence when I have been driving and sipping coffee on a number of occasions has caused my shirts to get familiar with Spray 'n Wash or a similar spot remover. When I have worn a dark shirt, it seems coffee never spills, but let me wear a light-colored shirt; my shirt becomes tainted. I started carrying an additional shirt just in case when I was working thirty-five miles from home. Damaged nerves in my lip/face from the previously mentioned accident could also provide an excuse for spillage of the java.

Different movements while working also provided an infrequent splitting of the crotch of my pants. This, too, caused me to take measures to have a pair of pants available in case an emergency occurred, and again when I worked at my second health agency. So I always had a new wardrobe available.

Just once, two odd things occurred simultaneously. I spilled coffee on my shirt in the morning, and in the afternoon when I bent over to take some soil out of the soil auger at a piece of property, my pants split. I changed my shirt in the morning and my pants in the afternoon. When I returned to the office, our secretary said, "You changed." I said, "No, I am the same guy I've always been."

Many times after we visited a piece of property, we would follow up the visit with a letter to the property owner or potential property owner. The mobile unit joker visited a lady's property who was deaf regarding placing in a new sewage system for her mobile home. Her daughter assisted in communications between him and the lady. When he returned to the office, he created a letter. Our secretary typed the letter.

It was tradition to end our letters with "If you have any questions, please call this office." Our secretary always included this closing statement, even if we did not include it when we composed the letter. Evidently the statement did not ring a bell with him when he reviewed the letter before it was sent out.

About a week later, he read the letter again and realized the statement was included in the letter. That afternoon he stopped at the lady's home and explained the error to her daughter and her when he was making his other calls. The lady and her daughter found it amusing.

In 1975 the additional workload induced our director to hire someone to assist our secretary. A very nice lady was hired to provide some support to our secretary. She held the position of clerk.

She lost her son in Vietnam. Our boss had known her husband and her for several years. She was a very innocent person. She was in her late fifties when she came to us. After working with her for a period of time, you began to realize she had a few quirks in her method of going through life and course of action regarding daily work procedures. She usually handled any person who came to our office to fill out any paperwork and also handled most of the phone calls.

She had a system of dealing with each client that she had memorized. If anyone interrupted her, whether it was on the phone or providing assistance to someone in person, she would start over and recite her memorized script. Sometimes this would irritate an individual, but most of the time her innocence would trump any impatience.

One time she told me that she and her husband had ten acres of strawberries. She asked if I wanted some for my family; she said she would give me some. I told her, "Sure, we would enjoy them." She brought in a saucer with five berries in it, wrapped in plastic wrap: two for me, two for my wife, one for my oldest daughter maybe. I did not fathom how I was to divide them up. She asked the next day if we enjoyed them. I told her we sure did. Maybe I expected too much; usually a quart container was applicable.

The lady clerk was a rather conservative person; long flowered dresses were her wardrobe of choice. So when she came to work one day in December 1978 wearing a gray pantsuit (a Christmas present from her daughter), we were surprised, to say the least.

The pantsuit became a need for further discussion when the suit was worn each day, I believe it was the first week in February when we started a lottery on when she would take a break for a day from wearing the suit. April 1 rolled around, and many of our projected days had come and gone. All the participants were on their second day of their proposed break in the wardrobe. One day in late April, the pantsuit was not worn, nor ever seen again. There was a rumor she might have caught on about the lottery, but we never knew for sure. Flowered dresses again were the norm for choice of daily work attire.

When our switchboard operator took her break, someone from the clerical staff would handle the board while she took this break. The staff took their turn on their assigned day. Our clerk was on the board one day when she received a call from someone requesting information regarding our division. She proceeded to go to her desk fifteen feet away. She answered the phone, "Environmental health." The information requested could have been supplied at the switchboard or transferred to our secretary, but again this would have broken her set work process. In the meantime, our secretary answered the switchboard until her return.

Another time I came into work and told her and others I had a dream the night before that we had rats in our basement (a result, probably, of working with rodent control at times as part of our job). For a couple of months, two or three times a week, she asked me if I had eradicated the rats. I would tell her each time it was a dream. Finally, when she asked, I just said yes, I did, and a short time later the questioning stopped.

Our boss said she was very sharp prior to her son dying in Vietnam. She did show signs of that at times, but other times, not so true, when her mindset was taken out of her routine or reasonable logic. She chose to leave the health department when our boss retired at the end of 1979.

I ran into her once in a while after that; she was always her cordial self. Every morning at work she would smile and say, "Well (your name), how are you today?" When I saw her after she left the department, she would again smile and say the same phrase.

In 1992 she developed cancer. She requested of her health care worker that I visit her, as she was terminal. I visited her a couple times prior to her death. We had an enjoyable conversation on both occasions. Every time I visited her she greeted me with, "Well, how are you today?" Her husband died a few months later. I understood it was mostly not being able to live without this caring, tender, and innocent lady.

There is a joke about a woman alone at her home while her husband is at work. It goes like this: Her husband's friend knocks on the door. She greets him. He in turn says, "Would you take your clothes off slowly and get naked for one hundred dollars?" At first she says no, then she thinks about it, realizing she could use the money for some items she has wanted. She proceeds to strip, and the friend gives her the hundred dollars. Her husband comes home after work and says, "Did George stop by and give you the hundred dollars he owed me?"

Repairmen, meter readers, and other service individuals have related stories of women they have encountered while visiting locations. Some of them I have found hard to believe, or they may be true, but they may have been embellished a trifle. On the other hand, I personally experienced some different fortunes. The fellow that took Racers job when he left came in one morning in 1977 and told us of a visit he had had the day before.

He was investigating a complaint that a woman and her child were living in a rental unit that did not meet housing regulations. When the woman answered the door, she invited him in. After his inspection of the premises and a short discussion, the woman asked him if he would like to go back to her bedroom, smoke some

Grass, and using her words, "Get it on." The woman was in her early twenties, about four foot nothing, was very obese and her hygiene practices left something to be desired, according his description of her.

I teased him through the years until he left the department in 1980. I really never was sure the story was true.

A few months before I left the department in 1989, I was covering an area for a girl who worked for me while she was on vacation. We received a complaint that a woman with four children was living in a mobile home that had unacceptable conditions. I did not check the name of the woman too closely until I arrived at the location. By chance the lady's name was the same as the woman my previous comrade had spoken of thirteen years before. The lady who answered the door fit the same description as he had indicated. I entered the home after she greeted me and inspected the interior and exterior, which had several discrepancies, including improper sewage disposal and cockroaches. After some discussion, the lady asked me if "she took care of my needs" (a new line), would I forget about the violations.

Neither my past coworker nor I ever cheated. The lady had four children, so someone must have gotten closer, than with a ten-foot pole; however, I would suspect that trying to bribe officials with sex was not embraced by an authority too often.

In 1975, I had two townships added to my workload to work in general services. In 1977, I received a complaint that a woman who lived in a mobile home park in my area had a leak in her plumbing that was noticeable from the outer portion of the unit.

One afternoon I visited the site. Indeed, the unit had water leaking from the front of the mobile home to halfway from the back of the unit. I found no one home. I visited the site at different times in the afternoon, finding no one present. I decided to visit the location prior to reporting to work one morning. I knocked on the door. A very attractive young woman answered the door in a nightgown. I stated my business. At first she said she was unaware of the leak. I then stepped down from the elevated step/platform and pointed out the areas of the leak. She said, "Oh yeah, I guess there is a little leak."

She placed her one foot on the rail of the platform. I, being on a lower level, saw London and saw France but saw no underpants. She then asked me if she could do anything for me. The remaining portion of our conversation was directed at her, but I was facing a direction away from her personage. I answered her question with, "You have forty-eight hours to repair the leak. I will return then to make certain the violation is corrected." She said, "I'll try, we'll see you, y'all come back now, you hear?" I told her I would return in two days to check on her compliance with my order.

I returned two days later. She was fully dressed that day, and the leak was repaired. No further discussion was made regarding "doing anything for me."

In 1987 I was again covering an area for one of my staff members. We had a request for a permit to replace a sewage system. When I visited the site, I knocked on the door. This was standard procedure. If we did not receive an answer, we proceeded to the area where the owner should have marked where the existing system was located. In some cases, we might have had a record of the system in the office if we had designed the original system. If this was not available or they could not find the system, we would search the property with a metal probe.

I did not receive an answer after knocking on the door. I therefore proceeded to travel to the backyard of the property. Walking between the home and the two-stall garage, I was met by a topless young woman. She had been sunbathing and had heard me knocking on her door, and had come to meet me.

She said "Oh the system is over there." She went back to sunbathing, She made no effort to cover herself. I could have had a free show; some men were at the time paying to participate in similar assemblies, but I chose to keep my back to her as much as possible and my eyes in a direction away from her while I was performing my investigation of soil conditions and the existing system.

I did ask a few questions about the plumbing inside the home. She did not act embarrassed, although I was little uncomfortable. She said she and her husband lived in the three-bedroom home, the number of bedrooms entered into our design criteria.

We had about ten structures that had been together, a motel in their day. Some said at one time they were part of a "no tell motel," but that was only a "roomer" (rumor).

These units were intended to be used by people who needed a place to stay while looking for another permanent rental unit. One week was the proposed duration of occupancy that was intended. Migrants who pick the crops in the fruit belt area stayed at the location many times when their grower did not have their housing ready. Social Services occasionally would use the location for emergency housing until they could find a place for individuals or families. Unfortunately, the combination of squatters and the owner trying to keep all units occupied caused these units to be rented for extended periods of time. Many times we were called to use our housing regulations to remove these individuals. Every so often we were called by someone to visit the location, and the parties would move on.

The facilities left something to be desired, to say the least. One time some poor traveler from Iowa had been traveling from the East coast from 5 a.m. until 9 p.m. Somehow he happened upon this place and decided, because he was tired, to stay. He called me the next day to complain. He said he stayed about one hour (why that long I do not know). I tried to explain that the place was not on the list of motels to stay in Michigan or the United States. He said the entire location ought to be condemned. I told him from time to time we did placard some of the units, but the owner fixed them up just enough to pass our liberal housing code.

The regulations of our housing code were too broad. Unless we had sewage on top of the ground or in the residence itself; unless they lacked drinking water or proper heat in the winter; or unless children were involved, the code was sometimes too open, allowing a landlord to correct violations by just getting by.

We attempted a number of times to upgrade the code, but getting it passed by all the governmental agencies that had a variety of types of housing in their area never came to fruition. This was also true at the second health agency I was employed.

One time a lady with six children was staying in one unit. Along with protective services, it did not take longer than a day to remedy that situation and get her into proper housing.

One day I received a call from the owner of the units; a man and woman had been occupying a unit for a month and had not paid him rent for three weeks.

I visited the location and knocked on the door of the unit in question. A slovenly man who additionally looked like many years of smoking had taking its toll on his entire body answered the door, buck naked. He stepped back, revealing in full view a woman who was also lacking any clothing about her person. She was pretty much in the same condition age-wise with the same body disrepair. Her breasts had seen a better day, and her nipples shared the proximity of her navel. In other words, both looked like they had been rode hard and put away wet.

The man said, "Oh, you caught us f***ing. I told him I would wait until he got dressed, but he said, "Suit yourself, but Cora and I don't mind talking to you now." I told him I preferred discussing issues regarding my visit with a clothed person.

He closed the door and returned outside the unit after putting his overalls on to discuss the reason for my visit. He said he did not want any trouble with the health department. He said he had had dealings with us on occasion in the past in our state and others and found us to be very helpful. He did not indicate for what.

He said they would be gone by sunset.

Sometime in late July or early August 1973, I was summoned to forty acres of property where a motorcycle group was spending weekends enjoying life together. The surrounding property owners in two subdivisions were concerned about having them as neighbors for the summer months.

A farmer in the area who had livestock (pigs and cows) and two hundred acres of land had endured a number of complaints from these individuals regarding the odor from his farm. He decided to lease forty acres of his land to this group. His answer to all those concerned was, "How you like them apples? You do not like my farming practices, so this will give you something else to think about." He said further, "They seem to be a nice bunch, and they have paid me an excellent amount of money to use my land."

I visited the site because basically they had all the requirements to meet the codes of that time period, but their food service process and garbage disposal was in question. The farmer was right; they were a little rough around the edges, but they were a cordial and fun-loving group. I will say I was a little apprehensive about meeting with the subjects, but once I began conversing with them, I was more at ease.

After they agreed to follow my suggested adjustments to their procedures while occupying the land, I left the property. The site continued to be a source of displeasure for the surrounding residents. They were not happy with our agency nor any police agencies; however, as long as they continued to comply with the regulations of the day, we could not make them exit the property.

Guidelines did get more stringent in time. The group did not return the next year, but the group did grace our area in 1977 on some lake property they purchased.

A complaint was received that the group was swimming in the nude, partying after midnight, and generally causing a nuisance on weekends. Jouster and the fellow who replaced Racer visited the site. They observed a few violations which could be easily corrected. They told them to swim in a more private manner and respect their neighbors with a curfew on loud interactions after sunset.

When looking around a bit, they discovered stacks of cases of Old Milwaukee's finest. Jouster and Racer's replacement were tempted to return that evening for further discussion of proper methods of consuming beer but thought better of it.

As they were leaving, they noticed a distraught horse who had seen better days. They asked what duty this poor nag could provide for them. They said, "Oh, we're going to roast her overnight Saturday for dinner on Sunday." Maybe that was why she had such a long face.

In the early years, health officials would find that equipment in food establishments had been installed in a manner that made it difficult to clean the equipment and surrounding area properly. As a result of these discrepancies, if the operators or their staff could not keep these areas clean, we would request the equipment to be changed to make cleaning it possible, or enclose it so dirt and grime would not come into play.

Some operators "balked" (remember, I learned that word early in my life) at doing this because of the expense; therefore, they would say they would try harder to clean these areas. Most of the time, their efforts were futile.

Among health-related concerns was also the possibility of fire danger around cooking equipment. Sometimes I was amazed that a grease fire did not occur in some places, when viewing the regions which needed attention. However, more times than not, a fire did not happen.

One time I was baffled, though. The operators of an establishment who were very meticulous about cleaning and whose equipment was installed properly had a fire at the bank of their cooking equipment. After investigation, it was discovered that a drip pan for the hood had been leaking a small amount of grease, which in turn had dripped on an electrical outlet and caused a short. Unfortunately, the location was closed at the time the shorting decided to occur, so there was appreciable damage. I felt sorry for the operators, because they tried hard to operate and keep a food service that met high standards of sanitation.

Speaking of fires, sometimes switchboard operators might give a call to an individual by mistake. On one occasion when I was director, I received a call by mistake that stopped me short for minute. The call went like this:

I said, "Hello," after the phone rang.

The caller said, "I am in a phone booth, and my pussy is on fire." I thought for a minute, gathered myself, and said, "I believe you wish to speak to our communicable disease section."

She said, "Okay, but I told you it is on fire, and it motherf____ing hurts"

I said, " I will transfer you."

The hurting part further assisted me in knowing that she did not have a cat who needed help, and the fire department did not need to be called.

The word motherf____er and other similar words have been used rather freely in the past two decades. Back in the decade of 1970 to 1980, it was used sparingly in my circles, but it was becoming more popular. Slang words for a woman's body parts such as "pussy" have also become commonplace in the vernacular of routine conservation. Again, in the aforementioned decade, these words were not used unless you were a bit uncouth.

I believe it was 1979 or somewhere around that time when I met a man at a piece of property who wanted to open a large restaurant and sizeable motel. After I told him what he needed to do and the possibility that he may need to reduce the size of his operations due to soil conditions, he said I was Mothef____ing government worker who had no idea what the real world was like. I proceeded to give him a condensed version of my background and life history. Sometimes this worked because it brought the angry person back to reality. Sometimes it did not. In conclusion, I told him that, indeed, I was married, had children, and did have relations with my wife on occasion.

This guy was big enough he could hunt a bear with a switch. Looking back, my shot at humor was a desperate attempt which could have worked or could have ticked him off even more. Luck was on my side this day. He began to laugh and calmed down. We further discussed his proposal, and he agreed to submit the necessary information and compromise his plan based on the restrictions of the property. The humor worked once, but I never tried the verbal comeback again. I still do not know what possessed me to make the "relations" comment.

I always told staff members that when we deal with the public we should realize that because we are a public official who has regulations and codes to enforce, whether a police officer or a health official, we put these people on edge. So you must understand, you may instigate a confrontational situation that you must handle with composure; appear unruffled, but not appear challenging, egotistical, or vain.

I followed up on a complaint once that took me to a residence where sewage was mentioned being atop the ground, and a man was using a stream behind his house for water. I visited the residence and knocked on the door; nobody answered after my three attempts at making contact with the occupant. I looked to my right about twenty feet where I observed that sewage had indeed gathered. I proceeded to go forward to take a closer look. As I took a couple steps toward my vehicle, a gentleman came out of the home. He yelled at me and said, "Who do think you are wandering around my property?" I identified myself, stated the reason for my visit, and I commented concerning my attempts to make contact by rapping on his door.

A debate over my right to inspect the area where sewage ponding was occurring later blended into a discussion about the horse manure laws that told him what he could and could not do on his property. He also said I had no idea what it was like to try to survive with limited resources of funds. He said he had three children and a wife to support. I told him I had the same. Comments were also made regarding government workers being a bunch of unconcerned individuals.

The conversation ended with me telling him I would follow up my visit with a letter that would state that he would be required to install a replacement sewage system, repair the existing water well, and we would have a hand in designing the sewage system. Furthermore, this letter would also indicate that he would need to make amends by a certain date.

He was a very upset man.

I visited the site with the "Boogermobile." It had been not starting on occasion; I had taken it to a repair shop three times, but they did not seem to be able to find the cause of my malady. This in mind, I carried jumper cables. When I entered the "mobile" and turned the key, it failed me. I had no alternative but to ask the fellow I had just ticked off to assist me. My inquiry for aid was met with, "What more do you want?" I stated my distressful development. At first he showed some uncertainty regarding helping me. Eventually he rescued me. A much different conversation ensued. Before I left, the gentleman conceded he understood now that I just had a job to do, and I had the same struggles he had in life.

I always felt when looking back at how the experience played out, if it had not been for my car not starting, my requested compliance date might have been met with more resistance, and he may have continued to have a bad feeling about government workers, specifically health officials.

I took the Boogermobile in again the next day to another auto service unit. There was a short in the line from the battery.

When someone died around Southwest Town during the 1950s, they were sometimes presented at the person's home, (which looking back, I find to be rather uncanny; however, that is the way it was done back than in many places). There was even a special door on some homes to bring the casket in and out. The door was usually constructed so the hearse could backup to the home and readily provide and retrieve the casket. We had such a door on the home my wife and I purchased in 1977. I changed the door in 2002, providing an exit to a deck I built off our house,

One person I knew took a picture of her husband in the casket and gave a copy to each of her late husband's and her brothers and sisters. We always said she could say, "Want see a picture of my dead husband?" if she carried one in her purse.

An older gentleman, who went to our church, was Irish and grew up in Chicago. Said when his uncle died during the 1920s, they had a traditional drinking gathering. After they had a few drinks, they decided to bring the corpse out of the casket and stand him up in the corner and have a few toasts.

This *Weekend at Bernie's* move may be frowned upon today.

When one of my uncles who never married died in 1955, my mother was helping my aunt clean the home of my uncle the township supervisor.

He was being presented there. My cousins, my aunt and uncle's children, decided to sneak up when no one was looking and touch his nose. We carefully plotted our strategy. One person would be the lookout while the other would casually graze the nose with his or her finger.

I was the first to complete the task without failure. Although I told the others it was rather creepy and not real exciting, the others chose to also have the experience of touching his nose. After the task was completed, all of us felt it was not an experience we cared to take part in again.

Some people like to go up to the casket and touch the deceased on the hand or the face, but to this day I still do not do so. After all, no matter how well the undertaker offers the viewing of the body, he or she is not "herself "or "himself" and has no feeling; he or she is dead.

The other option in the fifties was viewing at the funeral home, which soon replaced forever the home viewing.

The funeral home used by everyone in Southwest Town was in Southeast Town. A procession of cars always drove from the funeral home to the church in Southwest Town. My cousin who worked at the Oldsmobile plant lost his daughter to meningitis as a toddler, which was very sad.

My uncle the postmaster had to do some work at a house he and my aunt leased to others prior to the funeral. The funeral procession always went by this residence. My aunt did not feel well so she stayed home at the house they lived in. My cousin, their oldest son, dropped his dad off at the property and drove to the funeral home to leave word that his dad needed to be picked up. He needed their car to go to an appointment. When the procession went by my uncle's property, he was standing out by the road. My uncle waved and everyone waved back, a very cordial group; however, no one stopped.

Leaving my uncle by the side of the road was obviously caused because of a glitch in who was going to pick him up; the fault was never really determined. Also some pled that because the pallbearer's car was the lead car and was traveling much, much faster than a normal funeral procession should travel, trying to keep up with the lead car caused them to forget.

Sometime in the middle of the funeral proceedings, someone realized my uncle was not present. My Uncle was soon rescued.

Sometime around 1978 or 1979, I needed to take my car in for a tune-up. The day before the appointment, I asked Mobile Unit Jokester, since he was going by my house on the way to work, to pick me up at my house. The garage where I took the car was just down the street from our house. He said, "Why sure!"

I was waiting out by the road on the sidewalk by our house. My work buddy waved at me but did not stop. I waited a few minutes in case he got down the road and remembered. No such luck. I called the office. When he answered the phone he said, "Oh hi, Ger, what's up?"

I said, "Did you forget someone today?"

He said, "Oh, was that today?"

I said, "I was not counting cracks in the sidewalk when you went by."

He said, " I will be there in minute."

When he arrived to pick me up and I got in his car, he said, "Looks like you're going to be late for work; sorry Ger. I did forget, and when I answered the phone and heard it was you, I remembered and I knew I screwed up, but I did wave at you, and my wife says sometimes I am noticeably not very friendly in the morning."

Later in the morning, I related the story about my uncle to him, which came to mind after I thought about how both incidents were similar.

It has been said you can pick your friends, and you can pick your nose, but cannot pick your friend's nose. By the same token, you cannot always pick your neighbors, especially in a mobile home park. When we lived in the park in my college town, we had neighbors who took our charcoal for our grill. When they lost their unit because of lack of making payments, they were replaced with a fellow who sold drugs.

When we lived in the park we settled in when I took the job at my initial health agency, we had a married couple with a three-year-old boy who lived next to us in a westerly direction.

When you first move to an area where you do not know people, you accept situations and traits from people who live near you. We maintained off-again-on-again social contact with the aforementioned neighbors for about a year and a half. This type of relationship existed mainly because of the three-year-old boy, who was a hell-raiser from morning until night.

On one occasion he went into a neighbor's mobile home with two other children about the same age when they were not home. He took a loaded pistol out of their bedroom closet. The two other children said he shot the pistol. The shooter, whoever it was, shot a hole in the mobile home and the bullet also created a hole in the unit next door to that trailer and came to rest in that mobile home's dresser drawers.

The children took advantage of visits to the lady who lived there with her husband. The lady would invite them in to have snacks once in a while and play card games like Old Maid and Slapjack. Evidently at one time or another the children invaded the bedroom in question and discovered the pistol when the lady was not paying attention.

The boy was bold. When he would come over to visit my wife and our daughter with his mother, he would go from one room to another despite his mother's weak efforts to tell him not to do so. Once he came in and grabbed a chicken leg out of the refrigerator before anyone could stop him, took a bite out of it, and threw it on our kitchen table. Then he ran and grabbed a banana and took a bite out of that. Episodes like that caused us to ban him from our home.

This created uneasy conditions between these neighbors. Another child, a girl, came on the scene a year after we lived in the park. This child was a bit more under control, but still had the same tendency.

We were required to have skirting on our units. If this skirting was provided, an access door or opening was required to inspect the area under the unit to keep track of the plumbing and make certain any nuisance conditions, such as insects or harboring of rodents did not exist.

One day late in the month of May 1976, it was an unseasonably hot day. When I came home from work, I determined that an odor was coming from the bottom of our mobile home. When I removed the access unit piece, I discovered that the ninety-degree elbow that connected the mobile home to our sewer line had been cut with a device, and sewage had been gathering under our unit for some period of time. After some investigating, I found out that the now six-year-old boy was seen with his sister around our unit with a jackknife. A divorced woman was now attempting to raise the two siblings alone (a divorce caused as result of an affair the father had with the babysitter while the mother was working as a waitress). The informant stated that he did not know at the time what they had been doing.

It was embarrassing to me, being a health department official, to have an undiscovered sewer line unattached to my mobile home, a violation of codes. I cleaned it up immediately.

While I was cleaning it up, it brought back when my oldest daughter's diaper slipped out of my hand in 1972 when I was cleaning it and flushing the toilet at the same time. I crawled under the mobile unit, disconnected the elbow, and took a hanger to dislodge it. During the process and at the time the diaper was released, a shower was created-not a pleasant experience, to say the least.

When a basic sewage system was installed where municipal sewers were unavailable, in my early days of employment, a precast container of a certain size in gallons, depending the amount of individuals in the home was commonly placed in. This unit also had baffles at each end, the first to deflect any surging of sewage; the second baffle was to create a slow overflow movement of less thick liquid.

The idea of this "tank" was to allow for settling of sewage, allowing for the breakdown of sewage into a less thick liquid form. This flowed to a final disposal configuration which allowed this form of sewage to absorb into a soil that would drain well.

Three types of final disposal designs were fashionable: a precast dry well, a cement block-built dry well or a drainfield type that consisted of lines of perforated pipes. Stone was placed around the dry well units and around and under drainfields.

Drainfields were used when soils were not capable of providing an acceptable movement of liquid through these soils. Through the years, more diversified methods of sewage disposal have been developed.

Most of the time, these systems were installed by a contractor who had the equipment to readily place in the systems. Occasionally, a homeowner would place the system in. A drainfield installation could be a challenge for a novice.

Once in a blue moon in the early days, we would go out of our way to assist someone who was totally lost.

The gentleman that had the encounter with the lady and the bedroom visited a site four or five times to make a final inspection for approval to cover the system. Each time he visited the site, the lady and her young children who were attempting to place the system seemed to go backward instead of forward in succeeding to provide a successful installation.

One Saturday, I was his cohort in developing the drainfield correctly for the lady. It was a very hot and humid day. We had worked on the installation for about two hours. This length of time spent at this location had not been foreseen by us; therefore, we did not provide any refreshments for ourselves.

Two of the lady's children were playing nearby. These two shabbily dressed boys were sipping on a soda. Liquid matter was dripping from the nose of both.

Their mother said, "Why don't you boys give those hardworking fellers a sip of your pop?" As thirsty as we were, we still declined. We felt it was "snot" a good idea.

We were also offered egg salad sandwiches, which by their appearance came from a questionable source. Our method of postponing the partaking of these "delicacies" was to say, "Leave them; we will eat them when we get done here."

About forty-five minutes later we finished. During this time their dog came up and sniffed the sandwiches and retreated. A few minutes later, their two cats came up to investigate sampling of the "delights." They too were not impressed and turned away.

After we finished, we commenced to tell the lady of our finished product and tell her the system could now be placed in service. She interrupted us and asked us to now partake of her offerings. We told her we would take them with us.

There was a bar/restaurant a quarter of a mile down the road and around the corner. We stopped there to have lunch. Since my coworker drove to the site, I was "keeper of the treasures." I threw the sandwiches in the establishment's dumpster. I washed my hands thoroughly prior to indulging in my lunch order.

One of the school districts in the county that was centrally located offered a variety of evening classes. In the summer of 1973, I contacted the director of the program. We discussed offering a class for food establishment operators and the general public which would provide knowledge of proper handling of food and proper cleanliness. A certificate would be issued after completion of the class.

I could not put any mandatory tags on the class for operators because at the time there was no such requirement, so attendance was strictly voluntary.

The director of the program agreed to provide the classroom space and assist me in publicizing the class, which was to be held starting the third week in September 1973.

I worked extra hours at the office and at home developing the class materials and lecture substance prior to the first class deadline. I had discussions with operators regarding the class when I visited their establishment for inspections and sent out fliers to the locations I was not scheduled to visit. I placed announcements in local publications, and as I said, the program director also provided publications, which included a flier from his agency.

The night arrived. The time of the scheduled class was 7:00 p.m. I arrived at 6:00 p.m. with enormous anticipation and nervous energy. A number of operators had indicated they would be present at my class, which would consist of 4 one-and-a-half-hour sessions once a week. There was no charge for the class. Around 6:35 p.m., one gentleman arrived who I did not recognize, probably a person from the general public, I surmised. As 7:00 p.m. approached and no more people arrived, I thought, what am I going to do if this fellow is the only person who will be attending? Then about 6:55 p.m. the man who had sat quietly up till then said, "Is this the future grape growers class?" I waited until 7:20 p.m. gathered my things, and went home.

My wife consoled me. My coworkers were not so gentle. They found the incident rather humorous, especially the part about the gentlemen being in the wrong session.

I had many educational meetings which I conducted throughout the years; they were well attended. As time went on after that first attempt, I used it in various venues for a humorous anecdote.

A man who was my right-hand man at my second job location and I conducted several educational session together. We would share addressing the groups. We were very close friends as well. Our friendship worked as a huge advantage in conducting our daily tasks, which could be viable each day when something occurred like a food poisoning.

As result of our solid friendship, we would many times use humor to critique each presentation after we completed it. On one occasion, I pronounced "accolade" "accoloyd" when I said, "We just try to do our job of protecting the public. We do not expect any accolades along the way." This did not escape my friend. It continued to be a memento of periodic bantering.

On another occasion I used the 1950s word for footwear, "thongs," which now are known as flip-flops, to describe how a cook was dressed when I inspected a food establishment. I said. "The cook did not have a shirt on, only short pants and thongs." This raised a number of snickers, which I did not understand. After the presentation, my buddy explained that my choice of the word "thong" had been out of date. This, of course, remained as gaffe to be brought up at various times.

One of the reasons why I enjoyed the right-hand man's friendship was that he cared for others and would go the extra mile to help them.

However, one time we both got hooked in to helping someone perform a task. I use the word "hooked," because after we completed the task, we were left scratching our heads.

We visited a food service establishment which had been open previously, serving mainly ice cream products and a few types of sandwiches and French fries. The place had been closed for a few months. A new owner wished to reopen the unit. Right-hand Man and I were meeting the prospective owner to clarify what needed to be done to operate the establishment again.

While we were discussing some issues with the new owner, a gentlemen was present picking up a large, two-door refrigerator that the previous owner had evidently rented from his company. The new owner did not wish to continue a rental agreement, as she had her own equipment. He was alone and had only a less-than-adequate cart to gather the piece of equipment. We both watched him as we conversed with the new owner while wrestling with the unit. Finally he asked us to help him slide the unit to the door, where he had backed his truck up about twenty feet from the establishment.

There was very little assistance from the man. We mostly pushed and lifted the unit to his requested designation. Once we achieved that process, he asked us to further help him get it through the door and to the lift on the back of his truck. This procedure was accomplished with absolutely no effort on his part. The two mules performed this alone. Once we got the unit on the lift, he asked us to stand on the platform and keep it steady as he ran the lift. He than directed us from ground level to place the unit toward the front of his enclosed truck near some other equipment he had present and to furthermore secure the unit with some stretchable straps.

What put the icing on the cake was he never said thank you; he just jumped in the cab of the truck and took off. As we watched him drive away, we looked in amazement at each other, realizing that we had just been victims of a con job.

We always wondered what he would have done if we had not been present. We agreed that he was lucky the two pigeons flew in to assist him. (I use the term "assist" loosely.) We thought of sending him a bill.

Sometimes things are not as they appear to be. One night when Floyd, our dog, was young, a man came to our door. Without even saying hi, he said, "I got your G-Damn dog in my pickup I am tired of him being in my yard every night." I said, "You do not have my G-Damn dog in your vehicle; he is in our bedroom and has been there all night." He said, " Are you sure?" I asked Floyd to come out. He had been sleeping and came out, stretched and sniffed the man's shoes, and meandered back off our porch and back into the bedroom.

The man said, "I wonder whose dog I have in my pickup" I said, "I have no idea, but I wish you a lot of luck".

When someone suspects they have incurred food poisoning or that a food borne disease outbreak has possibly occurred, many people believe that the symptoms will begin soon after eating. In reality, only staphylococcus aureus shows signs one to six hours after the food item is consumed. All others do not show signs until eight to twelve hours and some days after eating food. As a result, many people suspect the last meal they consumed is the culprit.

We received a call from a doctor who said he had just treated a patient that had consumed home-canned beans. He said he felt we may be dealing with botulism. After interviewing the sixteen-year-old young man and his mother, I discovered he ate the entire contents of two jars of home-canned green beans in about a half hour. Botulism symptoms were not apparent, nor were any other types of food poisoning. After some encouragement, the mother admitted that her son was not supervised, and he had eaten a very large breakfast and an overabundant amount of food at lunch prior to his consumption of the jars of home-canned beans.

We had a mother call and say a school was serving spoiled potatoes. She said her daughter came home and said the potatoes served for lunch that day were green in color. Somehow the mother failed to realize it was St. Patrick's Day, and the lunchroom staff had used food coloring in the potatoes. When I brought this to her attention, the phone went dead.

I went to lunch one day at a restaurant where the owner kept a top-notch establishment; however, he liked to joke around. Many times he would ask the regulars, "Who ordered the dirty glass with your beverage?" or "Who ordered the fly in their soup?" or "Who ordered the hamburger with their mustard and ketchup?"

After I finished my grilled cheese sandwich and fries, I ordered a piece of my favorite pie, lemon pie. The owner said to his wife, "Do we still have that piece of lemon pie from two weeks ago that we were trying to get rid of?" Someone in the establishment heard this, and by the time I returned to the office we received a complaint that the owner was serving out-of-date pie, or "Pie a' la old". I called the fellow who was making the complaint. He commented that this had been his first visit to the establishment. I tried to explain the intended humor and that the owner meant no harm, but he did not seem to get the picture. He said if I was telling him the truth, he felt a licensed food operator should not be conducting himself in that manner. I politely told him the operator was a good operator, and most people liked his humor.

Watching someone fall on their butt seems to rank with men getting hit in the crotch. Many think it's funny, as long as you are not the one falling or having your privates struck. Falling on one occasion is one thing, but having it happen three times in three weeks, along with getting hit by a vehicle twice, is, to say the least, very unusual.

It began in mid-January in 2003. I had gone directly from home to my field visits. I made four stops and my last stop was at a food establishment located on a street in the center of several other businesses. The owner had a remodeling project he wanted to discuss. I finished our discussion, and as I approached my car, I did not see a small patch of ice on the pavement. In an instant I was on my back, hitting the back of my head, with paperwork flying in different directions. As I was gathering my papers and myself, I glanced around to see several customers walking and inside buildings, along with the business owners and their employees, laughing at my expense.

I was still a bit dazed as I arrived at the office. I discussed my damaged ego with a few of my coworkers, but they only cast more remarks about how they would have enjoyed watching my pratfall.

The following Monday arrived. It had snowed appreciably on Saturday and Sunday. I was about to cross the street, and my car was parked just around the corner. Suddenly a car came around this corner. Neither the driver of the car nor I could avoid making contact with each other. I grabbed the hood of the vehicle near the ornament that protruded. I slid several feet, skiing in a backward direction until the driver managed to bring the vehicle to a halt.

The driver was an older lady who became very apologetic. I was not injured, thank God, from the brief, thrilling winter recreation the snow-covered road had allowed me.. I spent some time calming the lady down; she was more shook up than me.

I had some sore muscles in my legs for a few days, which might have contributed to my next ordeal. The following Friday, I was in a walk-in cooler taking temperatures of two large containers of spaghetti on a tray.

As I moved backward, I slipped on the metal floor. The amazing thing is I landed in a sitting position and did not spill any portion of the product. My tailbone was a little sore, but other than that, no injuries were incurred.

The next Wednesday, I was again crossing the street in another town when a pickup truck came flying around the corner. I jumped back, but I grazed his fender. The driver stopped only momentarily to give me the middle finger and yell at me as to why I did not get out of the way. Again, I was not injured, but some bystanders were upset that the young man driving the vehicle did not stop at least to find out whether I was injured.

I did not tell any of my compadres at work of my contact with the older lady's car and my acrobat act with the spaghetti prior to the pickup truck run-in. The morning after my latest incident I did relate all three of my unusual occurrences to a number of my coworkers. Their response was somewhere between disbelief and shock. I quipped, "Maybe I should increase my life insurance policies."

Then two days later I was inspecting a ski lodge kitchen. There was about fifteen-by-five foot elevated slab located at the exit of the kitchen to the dining area. I took two steps on the slab and went feet-forward on my fanny. The manager said, "We have been wanting to place a rubber anti-slip mat here; you're not the first person to fall here."

The cement floor was not kind to my already bruised derriere. I had a hitch in my get-along for about a week.

That was my last so-called possible tragedy. At the time, the possibility of continued occurrences haunted me, and the lack of sympathy as evidenced by the caterwauling by others with each new experience made for a nervous three weeks and a few weeks that followed, wondering if something else would happen. However, these experience made fodder for future discussions about past occurrences.

I had hemorrhoid surgery in October of 1986. My surgeon told me I would need to be careful not to confuse passed gas with actual movement of the bowels.

One snowy morning in December of that same year, I was meeting a realtor at a home to take a water sample and evaluate the property for a proper water supply and sewage disposal. The realtor was late for the appointment because of the weather. As I was waiting, I noticed that my stomach was beginning to rumble. The driveway to the home advanced in a spiral and increased in elevation upward to the home from the road that brought you to the residence. I parked by the road.

When the realtor arrived, we had to walk through rough snow up the driveway. As I accomplished about half the climb, an expulsion came to pass as a result of my exertion from walking. What I hoped was gas soon became apparent to be a small gathering of fecal material. I proceeded to follow through with the evaluation. I do not think the lady realtor suspected anything.

When I returned to my vehicle, I luckily found two teen magazines which my oldest daughter had left in the car for some reason. I placed them on the car seat to protect the seat from any possible seepage through my underpants and jeans.

I had no further visits; however, the distance between the service and my home was appreciable, and I still had rumblings. The halfway point was a village where the courthouse for the county existed; the courthouse provided a restroom. In the restroom I relieved myself of my rumblings. However, I found it difficult to return my underwear to my body, so I placed my minimally stained trousers back on and wrapped my underwear in a paper towel and placed it in the covered waste receptacle. I returned to my car, drove to my home, took a shower, put on a new set of clothes, and returned to work.

The magazines must have been out of date, because my daughter did not inquire about them. My wife did question me about a missing pair of jockeys, but I told her she must have been mistaken. A couple years later, I related the truth to her

With this incident, I learned an extra wardrobe was advantageous, as I mentioned earlier. However, in 2006 I became less worrisome of any accidents or any other reason escapes me, why I failed to continue this lesson learn, I paid for it, literally.

I was inspecting a food service one morning, and when I bent over to look under a piece of equipment, the back of my pants split. I finished the inspection. The split at that moment was minimal; however, when I went to be seated in my low-rider car, the seam split even more.

I decided to stop at a party store/mart. I found they had some safety pins (one hundred count in a package). I went into their restroom, went in a stall, and a tried to enclose the gap, which by now was exposing my underpants rather freely. The effort was fruitless. Although my Fruit-of-the-Looms were hidden to a small degree, I still could not expect to carry out my duties for the day.

The nearest clothing store was not a place I normally shopped-they were a little pricey-but I had no other choice; any other store was much farther away. I drove to the store and purchased a pair of trousers for much more than I cared to pay. The safety pins are still in abundance. I made a necklace out of some of them once as part of a Halloween costume for a friend who dressed as Baby Huey.

Sometime in 1983, a woman that worked for me was having some problems with a food establishment, so we went together to the location to discuss the issues that were calcareous. After our meeting, she decided to stop at a residence where we had a complaint that sewage was running to a ditch in front of the home. The owner of the property spoke limited English, but his son was there to interpret our discussion. The woman who worked for me had completed two years of Spanish in high school and one year in college. Both individuals chose to speak to me because I was a man. I, however, had absolutely no ability to speak or understand the Spanish language.

The first part of the discussion centered on why we were there. The son said his father wished to know who had turned him in (much of the conversation was conducted with a smile on the father's face.) I told him I could not tell him, but he could inquire through the Freedom of Information process.

The son said his father said okay. (The "okay" response seemed longer.)

I told him that he would need to place an approved sewage system in.

The son said his father was reluctant to do so because he had raised ten children in the home with no problems from anyone, and the system worked. I explained that his idea of working was not the proper disposal of effluent from his home and was considered unhealthy.

The son said his father said he did not have the money to place the system in.

I told him I would be giving him a reasonable amount of time to get the money to make the corrections, but we could not grant too long a period of time to allow the violation to exist.

The son said his father said he would try to meet the requirements, but give him two months to comply. I told both of them we would follow up our visit with a letter, which would state the agreed-upon compliance date. I apologized for requiring him to spend his limited resources, but I had no choice. They both smiled and waved goodbye as we left.

When we returned to the woman's car and as we were driving, she told me the conversation was not as pleasant as it appeared. The father pretty much said he did not know why these government assholes were bothering him.

He said he was going to get the bastard who turned him in and they would be some sorry son of a bitches (a little more than the "okay" originally stated). He basically said it would be a cold day in hell before anything was done. He said he had the money to correct it, but we could get f____ed.

When I said we would be sending a follow up letter he said he would tear the piece of shit letter up.

When I said I was sorry for requiring him to make corrections he said just get off my f____ing land.

He said these things with, as I said, a smile on his face, and his son really did an excellent job of making the visit more cordial, to say the least.

Two and a half months later, after some further prodding, a new system was placed in. The person who installed the system and obtained the permit to place it in also disclosed that the woman who was responsible for the area where the home was located understood Spanish. This woman was the first woman ever hired with our department. I hired three others during the time I was supervisor, but this lady had a rough row to hoe for a time, as many women in our profession did during the 1970s.

I must tell a story about something that happened to her that was one of those situations that we all think happens only to us. The college that she attended had an occasional robbery outside the parameters, so you locked your car even when you went in to pay for your gas. Paying at the pump was not available at most locations yet.

One day we were out together on a visit, and she stopped to purchase a pop. We both went inside, and she locked the door. (This was also before keyless entry, so you manually locked the door.) I told her, "Someday you're going to forget and lock your keys in the car." She said, "It has never happened to me yet."

Suggestion many times causes things to happen. One day about a month after I said those words, she called the office and said she would be detained for a bit; she stopped to get gas and locked her keys in the car.

When God, according to the Bible, caused people to not understand each other, creating the first language barriers, history has proven that even different manners of speaking the same languages can cause misunderstandings. Saying the words, "Thanks a lot," can be interpreted in different ways. Saying those words can be found by the listener to be sincere or to be facetious, or can also be one saying that they object to someone's manner of treating the speaker, depending on the inflection of the voice.

We had a Spanish man working for the department at my second location who also spoke English rather well, but he did have somewhat of an accent.

Early on, when I first worked at the second department, we would tape our violation notices for our secretaries to listen to and type for sending out to our food establishment operators. This followed up on the handwritten report that was left with the operator and was a precursor to the laptop reports which followed a few years later. We used a canned unit of paperwork to specify the violation.

A "dipper well" is used to place scoops in for hand-dipped ice cream. It has continuous running water, which in principle is supposed to keep bacteria from growing. When our secretary listened to the tape of our Spanish employee, she heard the operator needed a "deeper well" meaning his water well needed to be made deeper. Unfortunately, the paperwork was sent out in this manner, and although our man explained this to the operator at the time of the inspection, he called me stating he did not understand the violation, since he did not have a water well; he had a municipal water source and had been hook up to it for five years.

Speaking of hand-dipping ice cream, someone called me one time and said a place was advertising hand-dipped ice cream: were they washing their hands prior to dipping ice cream? I told the person of proper handwashing procedures. After some further discussion, I realized she actually thought they were using their hands to dip the ice cream. That they were using a scoop in their hand I guess did not come to mind.

Supposedly a speakeasy, also called a blind pig, came into existence in 1888, when the Brook's High License Act raised the state's fee for saloon licenses from fifty to five hundred dollars in the state of Pennsylvania. The number of licensed bars plummeted, but many continued to operate illegally. A lady named Kate Hester had one such establishment for years in McKeesport, just outside of Pittsburgh. She refused to pay the fee and wanted to keep from drawing attention to her illegal business. When her customers got too rowdy, she would hush them by whispering, "Speak easy, boys! Speak easy!" This was further documented in a 1889 newspaper which stated that unlicensed saloons were known as "speak-easies." Of course from 1920-1933 during Prohibition days, all establishments that sold spirits were known as speak-easies.

In my time I inspected many, many bars or saloons. As might be expected, the more drinks most people had, the more "easier" it was to "speak" to a person of my calling. Many of these conversations were positive; many others were negative.

Negative comments were generally from those people who had an ax to grind about sometime when health officials and other authorities had caused them problems or made them spend money. Others had a bad feeling about all government authority and felt that our freedoms were taken away.

Most of the time, whether the discussion was positive or negative, I would try to just listen and comment only when asked a direct question.

However, on one occasion, I spoke to a man and listened to him and a very positive result came of it. The unfortunate thing, if there was one, was that I did remember having the conversation a few years later when the gentleman reiterated what the results were of my interaction with him.

Evidently he was sitting in a particular bar getting drunk, as he had in the past on a daily basis. I was sitting within earshot writing up a report. I was cordial to him, and we discussed different issues I guess, but only touched briefly on a major issue on his mind, suicide. The man could not remember exactly what I said to him about the subject because he was far along at getting drunk, but I said and did something that caused him to change his life. He said it was not so much what I said, but that I got up and went over and sat with him for a bit, which showed him someone cared about him. He also told me at the time that his wife was going to divorce him; his kids hated him; he lost his job because of his drinking; and had many other reasons for feeling despondent.

He told me this, as I said, a few years later when he was having breakfast in a restaurant I inspected. He told me he had quit drinking; he was still with his wife and kids; and was again working. I told him it was probably not just me, but someone else also. He commented that he and his family were going to church regularly.

Ryunosuke Satoro once wrote, "Individually, we are on drop. Together, we are an ocean."

Many times I found the characters that frequent these bars on a daily basis like to talk to someone else besides the *Cheers* locals. However, most of the time I tried to inspect early in the day for less hassle, and sometimes it was safer.

The first year of my vocation in life, I inspected a location which was frequented by some hard-living men. The owner was a retired marine drill sergeant. He had a baseball bat behind the bar, which gave me an idea what type of clientele enter his doors the first time I inspected it. The initial inspection did not in any way compare to my second visit. Upon this visit, which was close to 4:00 in the afternoon, some workers from an ironworks in the city had been drinking since about 1:30 p.m. There was great deal of one-up going on in some parts of the bar and some borderline heated discussions in other parts.

I was not listening to closely to the commentary, but as I went to back of the establishment to look at a storage container, I heard the owner say, "Take it outside you two." One of the individuals that he was speaking to then said to the other individual, "I'll be back you Motherf___er."

As I exited one of the restrooms I was inspecting, the man was returning with a butcher knife and stabbed the Mother___fer he had pointed out a few minutes prior. The weapon had been purchased at the hardware store adjacent to the bar. The assailant hovered over his victim for few seconds and than tore out of the bar. Police were called, and the victim was taken to the hospital. I left immediately and returned two days later, just after the owner opened, and went over the inspection with him. I found the owner to be a person who did not let things bother him; in fact, he said to me, "I hope you do not think that is the way it is in here every day." He laughed a laugh from the chest. "Sometimes it's worse."

The victim lived, and the assailant was soon after arrested.

On another occasion I had completed the inspection portion of a tavern and was writing up the paperwork to be completed. As I was doing so, two men were staring at me from a table nearby. Finally one of the gentlemen came over to me and said, "My partner and I like fat men." He suggested we might have a threesome sometime.

I told him I was happily married in a heterosexual relationship. He said, "Oh I am sorry; I must have read this situation wrong."

As I was driving away from the location, I contemplated how maybe their approach needed some work. Calling me fat was not very flattering; calling me portly or stout might have been a gentler proposal.

I was in a bar another time when a lady who was rather inebriated said to me, "I bet you could throw a mean f___". I said, "Excuse me." She repeated those words. I told her she would have to ask my wife.

I had a similar experience when inspecting an adult care facility. An older lady who no longer had all her marbles in her bag said, "I bet you have a big one in your trousers." The lady that ran the operations kept telling her to hush but she continued to follow me around stating her thoughts. When I left, she said, "You can come back any time honey." The operator was apologetic. I said I understood; visiting different venues, I had experienced many different situations in my time.

I heard someone question one time why the persons who serve you in sit-down food establishments are all the wait staff, when many times you, the customers, are the individuals who wait.

Two of my comrades at my second work location, one my right-hand man and another a young peer, and I would partake of lunch together at least once per week. They had voiced some concern with my lack of courtesy to those who served us. They said I did not thank the servers when they interacted with us when taking orders, bringing beverages, and food items, and follow up returns to our eating area.

One given day, we had rehashed my lack of politeness prior to our visit to an establishment we had chosen to obtain some vittles.

Our waitress was an older woman. She greeted us with a rather reserved attitude. She took our drink orders, and when she returned, I thanked her. I ordered the special, which was a macaroni-and-cheese and sausage concoction.

When she brought my order, I again thanked her. Once I took a bite of the entrée, I discovered it was cold. It took some time to flag her back to the table. When she did attend to me, she appeared to not take my request too kindly. My companions differed with my interpretation of her reactions to my petition.

In what seemed about ten minutes, she came back with my food. I said, "Thank you for your trouble." She just sort of grunted under her breath. When I took the first bite, it was cold again. My buddies got a big yuk out of that. I just ate most of the offering.

When she came back to our table, she asked, "How was everything?" I told her my order was still cold after she returned it to me. She said, "You are a big boy; you will get over it." My lunch companions found this to be hilarious, given the discussion that preceded this less-than-common episode.

I was very cordial to all wait personnel even after the aforementioned incident. Then about a year later, my two buddies accompanied me to another food establishment. Here I encountered another waitress with a glib attitude toward me.

She first got my order wrong; she gave me potato chips instead of the French fries I ordered with my hamburger. She acted put out that she had to order the fries. Then she more or less threw the fries at me when she returned with them. My friends told me that this time I should say something to her about her attitude. After I did so, they told her, "Don't mind him; he bitches about everything."

I heard a witticism one time about a man named Matt who bothered people so much that "Matt wore out his welcome mat."

Most times we received legitimate complaints that needed to be investigated; then there were those individuals who would contact us to complain time and time again about some concern that was unfounded or trivial.

A gentleman called our department at least twice per week for an extended period of time to complain about a particular restaurant where he said he became ill. He said he lived two blocks from the establishment, and by the time he reached his home, he developed diarrhea.

When he first called, we went through the standard interviews and field investigations, although he showed a reluctant attitude toward answering the questions we posed. We found little or no evidence that there were any problems at the food service unit that would cause him to become ill from the food served there. We also never received any calls from others that they became ill while eating at the location. After about the fourth or fifth call, we asked him why he continued to eat at the restaurant. He said, "Because the food is good." We suspended visits to the establishment after that. We soon just wrote his complaints off as a "Matt wearing out his welcome mat."

Another Matt-wearing-out-his-welcome-mat character was a restaurant owner who had an ax to grind with me because I had made him install a ventilation system for his pizza place. Every time he saw a new food establishment open or be remodeled, he would call me to ask me questions about what I made that business do before they were approved for construction. This went on for a number of years.

His son, who was about four years old when these conversations started, grew into a carbon copy of his father and even dressed similar to his dad. They both wore shorts even during the winter months and wore the same head gear each day, a baseball cap some days, other days a tam type.

One day when he was about ten years old, I visited the establishment to make a routine inspection. His son was the first person to greet me. He asked for my identification, even though he had known who I was for years. He then told me that his dad said I was an asshole. As I proceeded to conduct my inspection, his son informed two other employees, "This asshole is going to make an inspection of the place; try not to help him find any shit." When I completed the inspection, I went over the inspection with an employee and the man's son. As I was going out the door, the son said, "See you later asshole."

One of the employees evidently informed his dad of the manner in which his son spoke to me throughout the inspection. The next day the man called to apologize. After that, the man was a little more cordial, but he continued to call me every once in a while. Then one day he closed his establishment. I was told that he went bankrupt. Besides losing his restaurant, he lost his car and his home.

A legendary story among my peers in the environmental health field concerned the statement "See you later, asshole."

An environmental health director was known as a jester with a quick-triggered wit. Once a fellow asked him what he thought of his cowboy hat. Now the fellow who asked the question was a blowhard; basically he liked to try to flaunt his knowledge on any subject. The jester answered him with this quip, "It is like hemorrhoids: sooner or later every asshole has one."

The legendary quip involved the jester having a telephone conversation with a county official who was a Matt-wearing-out-his-welcome-mat type of individual who called the jester constantly about something. One day the jester had a conversation that involved much whining on the part of the official part.

After some time the conversation ended-that is what the jester thought anyway. When he hung up, he said, "See you later, asshole." The authority called back immediately, stating, "I heard you say something before you hung up. It sounded like you called me an asshole."

The jester said, "You heard wrong; I said see you later or so.

I guess the authority bought it.

The jester actually was one hardworking individual and one of the top leaders in our profession. He was also a great communicator with every person he came in contact with.

About a year after I completed my first year of employment at my initial job,

I found myself asked to perform a follow-up field training session with a consultant from our State Health Food Division. My boss said, "Your task, should you decide to accept it, is to spend two days with the state food gentleman." I said, " What if I choose to not accept it?" He said, "I would self-destruct in five minutes."

(*Mission Impossible* was still somewhat popular television show then, the reason for our banter.)

I had initially been trained by the same individual who was going to partake in the inspection training program. The man was a very nice fellow. He was a suit and tie type, a Ward Cleaver look-alike. By all indications he wore this clothing until he turned in at night.

I say this because once years later, I was visiting my cousin who lived in the same neighborhood as this man. My cousin received a call just before dark that his son was stranded with his car unable to start. We went to rescue him and passed by the gentleman's house. I glanced to my right and saw him sitting by his pool in his suit. I found this to be uncommon.

Our first visit was to an establishment owned by a retired marine sergeant. The cut of his hair was about as short as he could handle. He was a nature guy, the type of guy that walks through the woods swinging an ax, eating acorns and wild berries, hunting bear with a switch. He worked with combat boots on his feet and a belt on his Levi Strauss jeans with a big black horse buckle. He once told his idea of heaven was hunting something all day every day.

The state man's idea of heaven appeared to be going to a symphony; I believe bear hunting was the farthermost notion for him. I discussed wine making with grapes, watermelons and berries with him once. He said he did not drink alcohol, and he said he was allergic to strawberries. (I have made note of this not to disagree with either gentleman's lifestyle, but to put in perspective the contrast in their personalities that interacted during the inspection.)

Many local health department serfs agreed that when the state consultants performed evaluations or training sessions periodically, and they performed the actual inspection and followed up discussion of the issues found, they would be not as critical if they had to discuss the issues one-on-one with the operator. When they were under the gun, so to speak, they were willing to compromise. Many times they would leave it up to the local inspector to follow-up on the violation discussions at another time and expect stronger enforcement.

This date was no exception. The state official started out with about forty-five violations, and before he was done with the drill sergeant, they were reduced to about fifteen violations. Those remaining were listed as recommendations with a basic slap-on-the-wrist attitude.

This was agreed upon after an hour-and-a-half discussion with the conclusion that I would not find any of the violations and recommendations in the future, nor would they be tolerated. This gave the appearance to me that it took the heat off the consultant and placed it on me.

When I returned for the next inspection the operator stated, "Your buddy kind of hung you out to dry. I hope I was not too hard on him."

The next inspection was at an establishment that had a record of good operations in the past. The operator ran a grocery/bar establishment with limited food preparation. The operator was an older lady who indicated that she had grandchildren older than I was. She was a stickler for cleanliness. She was mopping the floor in the grocery at the time of our inspection.

The consultant and I went outside the establishment to conduct an evaluation of the dumpster, the water well, the onsite sewage disposal system, and other details. It had been raining for about two days straight. I managed to clean my shoes prior to re-entering the establishment on the mats in the vestibule. My friend from the state was wearing boots over his shoes, and for whatever reason did not manage to remove these boots or at least try to remove the dirt particles on the appropriate mat prior to re-entry. He then proceeded to walk over the just-mopped area.

The lady nailed him. She said, "Young man, you march yourself right out that the door and take those boots off, and when you return, do not walk over my wet floor."

The error in judgment reduced his authority a bit. When he discussed the few issues with her, which she corrected immediately, the lady did not relax her attitude. She said, "Young man, you got a lot to learn about your job. You two boys both need some more training."

I wanted to tell my state friend afterward that I took the bullet with him for his lack of good judgment. But I remained mute. He did not comment any further regarding the incident.

The next day went better, although I was the one conducting the interviews after we each conducted an inspection and compared our findings. I passed the training session after a number of comments on how I could make improvements in my method of inspection and interviews.

The state man did leave me with two reflections. The first was, "What will matter in life and your job is what you learn and how you use it." The second was, "Teach first (educate); enforce as a last resort. When a food service operator and his staff get in the habit of following the right procedures daily, they and you can expect good results." I continued to follow those words of advice and tried to impress others to also do the same.

A few months after I became director at my first job location, I hired a gentleman who turned out to be a born-again Christian. Every day, if he stayed in the office for lunch, he would read the Bible. He would become so in enthralled in his reading that sometimes I would need to remind him that his lunch period had expired.

He wrote others and me a note saying he found our language hurtful to God.

He told me that at one time he used such language, but now that he was saved, he found such manner of expressing one's self to be unacceptable. He furthermore said that all who used such words were not going to be accepted in the kingdom of the Lord. I told him I agreed with him and told him the story of my father's encounter with the man who worked in our cornfield. However, I told him I did need to clean up my language and would try, but sometimes words would slip out, and that I beg the Lord's forgiveness for doing so, and that we all were sinners.

Another gentleman who worked for me told me he did not get one of the notes; he said maybe the fellow felt he was beyond saving. One time the Christian man and I were out the field following up on a concern he had with a piece of property which he wanted my advice in handling.

The muffler on his car came loose and began to drag. He got out of the car and used some pretty harsh words that he had fought against saying. The door was closed, so I guess the noise level caused by the unattached muffler made him believe that I did not hear him. At least he did not act guilty. He left our department a year and a half after his initial employment to become a missionary for his church.

The size of my head has been considered to be a point of discussion throughout my life by many. An eight-and-a-half-inch hat size has doomed me to search more than usual for a head covering.

I was rather on the thin side for my six-foot, four-inch height all my life until I married, something that has not been an issue ever since. In fact, the opposite end of the spectrum has grown with age.

When anyone observes a photo of me in my younger days, they make comments such as: it must have put a strain on the other parts of your body carrying that melon around; or, how did you manage to keep your head up when someone said heads up?; or, did your head weigh more than your body in those days?

In the county I first worked there was a man who was a German citizen and became an American citizen. This gentleman owned and operated a campground which also had a motorcycle and dirt bike racing venue. When he first developed the business, he tried to sponsor a concert for country music fans, with local country bands providing the music on his property. He expected five thousand people to attend. This was in 1979, when these types of festivals were a carryover from the days of Woodstock.

Another gentleman from our office and I met with the owner to discuss the health implications and requirements. The other official and I were discussing the number of portable toilets that needed to be supplied for this function. We were a distance away from the owner but evidently close enough for him to hear our conversation. I commented to the official that I did not feel we could provide the answer to the owner until we returned to the office to use the formula we had for calculating the number based on the number of estimated attendees. My friend said, "You mean you do not have the answer bouncing 'round in that big head of yours?"

The owner evidently only heard the "big head" comment and asked, "Is there a requirement on the size of the Port-A-John? I thought they were all the same size."

I said, "No, he was commenting about something else." I did not further address the comment but chose to explain a number of other requirements that still needed to be pointed out. The gentleman had a dry sense of humor.

A few country songs in those days were recorded about hitchhiking down South and riding in trucks and cars with dead country music stars for a number of miles. With that as a theme I guess, the campground owner told me once, tongue in cheek, that when he was younger and first came to this country, he hitchhiked down South hoping a country star, dead or live, would pick him up. He smiled and chuckled after telling this tale.

With this in mind, I was not sure that this guy was not pulling my leg about the big head comment, or, whether he was serious in this regard. At times there were misunderstandings because of a language barrier regarding understanding his word processing and him understanding my communications, so he could have been sincere. I was also not sure if the word "head" was in his vocabulary for another name for a toilet or restroom.

As I said, my head has been the target of much humor over the years.

My middle daughter, on one occasion at a gathering, said, "Dad received some awards at his work, but he never got a big head, because he already had one." In addition, a friend of mine, when considering the possible purchase of a sweater for me as a Christmas present, said, "Better buy one with a loose collar so he can get his big head through it, or it will get stuck."

My body, as I mentioned, caught up with me a bit and expanded throughout the years.

One night my body and head became a so-called weapon. This particular night began when my wife and I attended an office Christmas party for the group from my first work location. We had an enjoyable meal at a local restaurant. The entertainment however, was a one-man band who I hoped had a day job outside of entertainment.

My wife and I decided, with two other couples, to adjourn to another restaurant/bar nearby which had a live band where we could enjoy the music, have a few drinks, and dance. A short time after we sat down, a man sat behind our table on a barstool.

Because I had a supervisor's position I wore a three-pieced suit to the party, so I may have been a little overdressed for the bar crowd. The man on the barstool kept noticeably staring at me to a point that we all questioned what was his problem. I got up to traverse to the restroom. He followed me in the room. When I finished my purpose of being present, I washed my hands. As I turned to leave the man said to me, "Did your mommy dress you tonight?" I tried to ignore him, but as I walked away, he tried to shove me. Unfortunately, he was about eighty pounds lighter and about ten inches shorter than I was. When I pushed back, he tried to grab my head. I just straightened up more, and with a shoulder shiver from me, he landed in the long urinal that could be used by three to four people at a time. I continued out the door of the restroom. I provided no assistance to help him out of the plight he brought on himself.

As I returned to our table and proceeded to sit down, we witnessed him exiting the restroom and leaving the establishment. We never saw him again. After he was gone awhile, we discussed the possibility of him going home to someone with wet clothes that had the essence of urine on them.

My second-hand man at my second location and I were heading for a two-and-one-half-day training conference a 2½-hour travel distance from our homes. We had traveled for about a half hour when I suddenly had the urge to eliminate some waste from my bowels.

My fellow traveler was operating the vehicle. I informed him of my plight. Unfortunately, he did not wish to stop immediately so I could take care of my needs.

After about another half hour, the urge advanced to an emergency condition. My groaning from the cramping in my stomach brought a mischievous smile to my partner's face.

Finally after fifteen more minutes, an exit off the expressway we were traveling brought a McDonalds Restaurant into play for a means to relieve my discomfort. I rushed into the restroom, sat down on the royal throne, and immediately, with little resistance from my body's natural functions removed my distress. However, when I took action to complete the process with the use of toilet tissue, I discovered the tissue was no longer available. The evacuation area lacked a door for privacy. However, both sides had a wall that existed about halfway from the floor to the ceiling.

I stood up and found over the wall to my right an available paper towel dispenser within my reach. This material was not the kindest surface to be applied to a sensitive area of one's body, nor was it appropriate for traveling through the plumbing. I had no alternative, though, but to make the application.

When I left the restroom and approached where my friend was sitting, I noticed he was laughing with great pleasure. As I sat down, he said, "You poor guy, first I make you wait, then I noticed from my angle as someone opened the door to the restroom a hand reaching over the wall to grasp the handle of the paper towel dispenser. You sure have the luck."

I reciprocated by saying, "The paper was bad luck; your not stopping soon after I asked was just you being an ass, and had nothing to do with hard luck. Some day the shoe will be on the other foot." About a year later, my prediction came to pass.

My subordinate and I were traveling to another conference; I was driving this time. When we reached about forty miles from our destination, my companion made the mistake of informing me that he had to pee. As a result of this comment, I decreased my speed considerably. After about ten minutes, my friend said, "Oh, I see what is happening." I just smiled.

When we reached the destination, I made sure I parked as far away as possible from the check in desk of the motel where we were staying, with the thoughts that a restroom probably would not be close either. We needed to walk a considerable distance. His gait, needless to say, was quick but uncomfortable. I told him paybacks are hell.

The curious part was, where I parked ended up right in front of the door to our room, therefore we did not need to carry our luggage far after we registered. I did not predict that.

I enjoy watching sporting events, both attending such events or watching them on the unit where cameras are present and commentators are available to describe action and nonactions. More and more it appears that we need people to explain to us what is going to happen or what just happened. As time goes by, nonaction is becoming more and more fashionable. We sports fans seemingly need to be delivered ceaseless information they feel only they know or only they are aware of.

We need to be told why, when, and how a back door, side door, or front door fastball should be thrown in a baseball game. The arm slot from which a pitcher throws must be cussed and discussed continuously.

Endless opinions must be given on decisions and talent levels by football players, baseball players, hockey player, golfers, basketball players, managers, coaches and just about anyone connected with sports. This endless chatter has replaced the unembellished commentary of an Ernie Harwell broadcast technique. Commercials have also attributed to nonaction. Television timeouts have assisted basketball coaches at times to stop a rally or attempt to stop the momentum of a team.

Some individuals, including my wife, have commented that sporting events such as baseball and golf have more nonaction than action. They say that watching grass grow and watching fish swim in an aquarium is more exciting than watching these sports. This nonaction has made high school sports events more pleasurable to attend and to follow the more continued action.

Well! That was my momentary pause for an editorial.

Basketball, for many years after I left my high school days, continued to be my sport of participation until my fifty-second year of age. A gathering of a group of fellows every week on Wednesdays during late fall, winter, and early spring seasons met at an elementary school, which provided some exercise and contact of a basketball with the hoops in the small gym available for us to play in during the late 1990s and early 2000s.

Contact with the net became less frequent as I aged. The aging process seemed to cause the touch of my fingers to the basketball to be less serving to the scoring process and less able to obtain instant gathering of the ball after an errant shot.

My right-hand man and I were on the same three-on-three or four-on-four team rather often. As the years went by, it became more frequent, because when grouping for teams occurred I was more of a liability, therefore my minion would join me in opposing other teams-out of friendship, I guess. An occasional spark of a number of successful attempts such as shots from the side and the key area, however, would provide mutterings from opponents regarding how I never shot that well when I was on their team.

My position was normally near the goal, because, for one, I am six foot, four inches tall and have less-than-average ability to bring the round ball down the court. We played first team to ten the winners, each basket one point.

Many discussions on breaks at work after a night of competition was centered around my minion's lack of passing the rock to other gentlemen on his team who might be available for placing the ball in the hoop closer to said goal. When the defense would guard him farthermost distance from the basket, he would fire up rainbows that most times would be unsuccessful. We discussed the possibility of working the ball in more, in order to have another teammate attempt a higher percentage shot and avoid the high trajectory from his bricks. The consequence of his bricks made offense rebounding less possible for those who were positioned near the basket.

When confronted with my concerns, my friend would answer with a sly grin, "I was open for the shot. Besides, you taller dudes should be able to rebound my shot, then you can place the ball in the hoop if I miss, and I also do drive on occasion." His "driving to the hoop" provided the most interesting deformities of facial expressions equating to a Halloween mask. Sometimes a successful score was registered, but more frequently the connection through the net was incomplete. A few times the bottom of the rim coming in contact with the ball created an in-your-face, literally, projectile. An unsuccessful score would cause a "Nice move ex-lax," comment. Actually, these types of barbs were exchanged frequently and were part of the enjoyment of participating.

I should denote here, however, that we did win a few contests every night, and my coworker had his hand in all our conquests.

Sometime between my thirty-ninth and fortieth birthday, I became a steady participant in the game of golf. Chasing a ball around a cow pasture, as some have commented regarding the game has become my favorite sport to this day. On one occasion my right-hand man and I met after work to play a nine-hole course. When we proceeded to pay for our round, my partner discovered he had not brought his wallet with him. I assured him that I would cover his fee.

He proceeded to beat me by large margin. It was a very hot day. I commented as we returned our clubs to our vehicles that I hoped after the thrashing he gave me he was not thirsty, because I was not about to bail him out for a drink. I did, however, a short time later, after my intended humorous comment received a guffaw from my friend, buy lemonade for him.

I never have enjoyed gambling very much; I hold my money to close to my vest. I have, however played nickle dime poker games on occasion here and there.

One particular night, I chose to join a poker game that was at a residence twenty-five miles from my home and thirty miles from jokesters home. Jokester and I traveled together to the site of the game of chance. Amber fluid (beer) was brought to the site by each participant and also served.

I was designated driver, so I did not take part in the consumption of this adult beverage. Even though 95 percent of the participants had to go to work the next day, the game lasted until 4:00 a.m.

The terms "just one hand" and "just one more beer" became steady commentary from about 1:00 a.m. on. Every choice of game played I believe was chosen at least once throughout the night, including a final winner-take-all game of Indian Shithead. Anyone who has played the game knows that you are dealt one card down, then you place the card on your forehead without looking at it. Everyone knows your card but you, and you bet on your card or not.

On the trip home about halfway to Jokester's home, in the middle of a residential area where no barns or stables existed for at least five miles in any direction, a horse ran across our path in the road home. The animal was close enough for me to need to apply the brakes quickly.

At first I thought my lack of sleep had caused me to hallucinate, but my friend soon said, "Wasn't that a horse?" I said, "What is a horse doing in this area?" We continued on our way home and did not comment any more. Needing to be at work at 8:00 a.m. provided minimal rest.

I was tired and Jokester was tired once we arrived at work. Another gentleman from work who had also attended the gathering was also dragging. The consumption of an appreciable amount of orange juice was being performed to soothe the effects of the night and morning before.

A discussion of the horse we had witnessed was brought up as the morning progressed. Several individuals made comments with a variety of interpretation, mainly centering around how much Jokester and I had had to drink and furthermore questioning our sanity. Adding to the lack of credibility to our tale was that no information ever became available through the gossip mill or through the media that a horse had been seen at the location, nor was one found to be missing from a site.

This occurrence became a constant source of mockery for a extended period of time. "Seen any horses lately? " Seen any horse's asses lately?"; "Played poker lately that made you see things?"; and "Roy Rogers was looking for Trigger; you seen him?" were comments made.

A longstanding summer function that has continued to be conducted in the rural setting is a county fair. This production has served as entertainment for the young and old. It also has provided a means of leadership and responsibility for the youth who enter their specific project or projects for judging purposes. In many cases, the raising of animals for judging purposes has taught and caused boys and girls to give their attention to something besides a computer game or the latest electronic device.

It has been stated, "Give a child a fish to eat and he will eat for one day. You teach a child to use a computer, and he will play games for hours and even several days straight."

Most fairs have cotton candy, French fries, candy apples, elephant ears, sausage and other food items; these have been available for many years. Also, most fairs have display booths, games of chance, musical entertainment, and amusement rides for young children, teenagers, and adults. A day at the fair can dig deep into one's pockets but is an experience still enjoyed by most people. Taking your best girl to the fair or walking around with your buddies trying to look confident and serene still is the order for the teenager.

The fairgrounds for the county I lived in was located within walking distance of the office of my first health agency employment stop. Therefore, during fair week, employees would spend their lunchtime alleviating their hunger by purchasing food items from one of the food vendors.

On one occasion, three of my coworkers and I visited a unit that served sausages for the main item with some additional items. When I stated my order, I told the man who waited on me exactly what I wanted on my sausage and also ordered French fries and a medium lemonade.

Prior to the placement of my order, another customer requested an item the unit did not serve. The man was rather rude to this person and said, "Can't you read the menu board?" He, however, said to me after I placed my order, "Now this guy knows our menu. He could work here." This resulted in rumors that I was going to quit my job and join the traveling carnival.

Two days later a going-away luncheon was held. A chef's hat, an apron, and several cooking utensils were provided by some of the staff at our department to use in my endeavors.

A card was signed with messages such as "We will miss you"; "Local health official takes an advancement in his career"; " Write when you can when you get a break"; "I hope you're not making any concessions."

The hoax was more entertaining than when I actually left the department a few years later. My luncheon was to be on my last day, but I was summoned to testify in a court case at the last minute, and it could not be postponed because I was starting my new job the next day. I ate the leftovers; I understand those who attended enjoyed themselves in my absences. My boss gave a little speech in the afternoon to some of the employees who went on break in my regard, but that send-off paled in comparison to the hoax gathering.

"Tuna fish or butter, tuna fish or butter" was a declaration I heard from one particular lunch lady from my first year of education to late in my third year. The words echoed throughout the cafeteria each day as you waited in line to be served and throughout the time that you consumed your libations and provisions. The quick manner of expressing this verbiage along with a German accent caused her to sound like she was saying "tuner fisher" or "butt her." If it was not enough to hear this every day during lunch period, it was also popular to mimic her on occasions when humorous banter was exchanged.

I attended the lunchroom for my specific school for twelve years. During these years, I remember you could have all the butter sandwiches you wished. Baked beans were also in abundance on Mondays, Wednesdays, and Friday. I took advantage of this benefit by combining these two items for butter and beans sandwiches. This combination grossed out some people. My friends said I did not need gas for our family car; I could provide all of the gas we needed. However, I do not recall having any major expulsions as a result.

It has been recorded that the very rich and nobility were the only individuals who were educated in the entire Western world for a few centuries. Then the Catholic church championed the introduction of education for the common man. The Catholic church's pioneering role in universal education opened the door for other private schools to guide the youth in academics. When I was young, the close proximity of some type of school was readily available. As the 1960s and 1970s became history, these schools were reduced for different reasons, lack of funds being one reason, and consolidation being another.

When I began work at my first position, there were five Catholic schools and one Lutheran school in the county. Private schools still exist today on a small scale. One day sometime in 1990, I was inspecting the cafeteria of one of these schools for the second time. After checking out several locations, I realized I had forgotten where the cleaning of dishes and utensils used in preparations and service was being conducted. I thought I remembered a mechanical dishwasher being present at the location. I asked the supervisor where the dishwasher was. She answered by saying, "In the basement."

I proceeded to take a trip to the basement, believing I was going to observe a mechanical unit. I was greeted by a gentleman who I asked where the dishwasher was located. He responded, "I'm it," and proceeded to direct me to the three-compartment sink where he performed the necessary tasks.

My misguided belief that a mechanical unit existed and the statement "in the basement" by the supervisor further contributed to my misconception. Sometimes circumstances fall into place that result in misunderstandings that become humorous.

Coffee is believed to originate in the Kaffa region of Ethiopia, which gave the drink its name. It evidently spread to the Middle East, then to Europe and henceforth throughout the world. After oil it is the world's most actively traded commodity. It passes through the hands of middlemen several times and is resold several times. As a result the farmer who produces it does not get much money for his product.

I guess what coffee one purchases to consume is the "Taster's Choice"

A health inspector is encouraged not to take gratuities from any person they come in contact with when enforcing laws and regulations. However, coffee is acceptable to provide a comfortable means of discussing issues.

Teddy Roosevelt said when addressing the subject of laws, "No man is above the law and no man is below it; nor do we ask any man's permission when we ask him to obey it. Obedience to the law is demanded as a right; not asked as a favor." However, I believe in most cases when developing enforcement procedures, a little sugar will work much better than vinegar. The inspector has within his structure to be hardnosed, as Mr. Roosevelt insinuated.

When a group or an individual chooses to not comply in a proper amount of time, the sugar will become acidic. Sometimes, as noted prior, too much coffee can cause certain individuals to become more aggressive and be less given to listen carefully to what others are saying. This occurred several times to those who worked for me and with me, as well as for me personally.

Such was the case when I met up with a restaurant owner one day. This gentleman informed me when I arrived to perform an inspection of his establishment that he had consumed an appreciable amount of java throughout the day since 6:00 a.m. It was 3:30 p.m. when I arrived.

By nature the owner was somewhat a bit of an enigma as per his personality; along with being a bundle of nerves, the coffee only created a less stable person. I began my inspection after my normal introduction, which he had gone through a number of times with me earlier. He followed me around like a two-week-old puppy, basically being underfoot with my every move, sipping on a cup of coffee as we traversed through the establishment.

"What are you looking at now?" "Why are you looking at that so intensely?" He asked his continuous questions. I would give him a short explanation and assure him that I would discuss any issues when my inspection was complete.

After I completed the inspection, we sat down at a table to discuss the results. There were a few items to be gone over, but overall the establishment had a history of limited violations.

The first two items of discussion were accepted with agreement; however, when I noted that the salamander needed more attention, before I could explain the exact portion of the unit that need cleaning, the operator went ballistic. He began yelling that he did not have any animals in his establishment. Furthermore, he said, "Where did you see this salamander, and have you lost your mind requesting it be cleaned and not be removed from the establishment?"

It took all my abilities to refrain from laughing. If it had been anyone else, I would have thought he was trying to be funny, but I realized he was a no-nonsense man, and his set jaw also trumped any notion of humor. I said, "Hold on a minute; let me explain." I asked him to follow me to the location of the portable warming oven. He said, "Oh, you mean the browning oven. That's a salamander?" I proceeded to show him the areas that needed cleaning.

The operator never apologized for his gaff. I could not come up with any explanation other than his abundance of coffee caused him not to think straight; or along with the coffee, he was nervous because of my presence. Whatever it was, the whole experience was an enigma in itself.

We have not always treated our elderly the best, for a number of years. In other countries when a mother or father are older and need assistance, they are welcomed into the home of one of their children, not as a subservient but as an equal or as an elder advisor. In that regard, children in this country often move back home after graduation from high school or college and want to rule the roost.

I knew a married couple during my first years as a health official who had owned and operated a successful restaurant for years since the 1940s. They were in their early seventies at that time. They were known to give others a free meal occasionally if they were in need. They were particularly partial to college students. They also helped families throughout their community. They were a benevolent couple. They were the true "Ma and Pa" restaurant by definition. They served a quality breakfast and lunch. They were not open for the dinner crowd. In the summer, the tourists added to their normal daily clientele, and in the winter, the growers spent many hours eating breakfast or just drinking coffee while shooting the bull.

However, the mid1970s gave way to fewer customers because of fewer small farms, and more competition from other food establishments became a reality, causing people to not visit them as frequently as they had before. Their age also slowed down their time of service to the customer. Fast-food service had entered their world.

In May of 1976 the wife developed cancer. The man's attempt at trying to tend to her needs and trying to keep up with the operations of the restaurant caused the business to suffer. As a result of giving so much to others, their bank accounts had little or no funds. The woman's medical bills and the lack of business took its toll on them and they struggled with paying their bills for supplies, utilities, upkeep, and other expenses due for the establishment.

At least once or twice a month, I would stop in their establishment for a late lunch if I was in the area. The man and his wife were wonderful people. I would discuss a variety of subjects. He was originally from Pittsburg, Pennsylvania. He loved the Pittsburg Steelers football team and loved Art Rooney. He said he suffered through many losing seasons with the Rooneys as the owners for years, and now the Rooneys and their fans were being rewarded. He always said Art Rooney was the most popular owner in all sports venues throughout the nation. He was finally rewarded in 1975 and 1976; he loved talking about each player.

He was evidently born in Denmark, and his folks moved to this country when he was small. They became U.S. citizens soon after. He always called himself a Jutlander because he said that was where his folks immigrated from. He explained that it was a peninsula in northern Denmark where some battle was fought early in the 1900s between the Germans and the British. He had a rather lengthy description regarding his personal interest in the area and the battle, most of which I do not remember. I did some research regarding it, and the battle indeed occurred in 1916. I never heard the term "Jutlander" before he discussed it with me or any time after.

One day in July 1977, I stopped in just a bit before their closing time of 2:00 p.m. I ordered a vanilla shake. I asked the man, "How is your business?" He said he made seventy-eight cents all day. He brought the shake and sat down to discuss the latest issues of the day. He then got tears in his eyes as he informed me that he may need to close the establishment; he could no longer afford to stay open.

When I went to leave, he told me the shake was on him. The shake cost eighty-two cents. I left two dollars on the table. As I was getting in my car, he came running with the money. He insisted he would not take the money. He said he would be insulted if I paid the bill, and he would never speak to me again. Just before Labor Day that year they closed. Many people were upset that they closed, however they did not close because people were visiting the location.

The conveniences of fast food outweighed helping them out during their troubled times. I heard they moved to live with one of their children. I never saw them again. I heard through others that the woman recovered, but the man died a few years later after developing a form of dementia. Others said they thought he died of a broken heart. I always wondered if he lived long enough to witness or realize his beloved Steelers winning the SuperBowl 1979 and 1980.

The day the man gave me the shake always stood out in my memory, the day he gave away more than his profits for the day. Some would say nice people finish last, but I think this man and his wife finished first in many respects that are an important part of living for others.

One very snowy and slippery afternoon, I was following a car and its driver traveling about twenty to twenty-five miles per hour. I had appointments for work to fulfill in a number of locations. I could see that the driver was holding on rather tightly to the steering wheel; I could just imagine from the position of her hands on the wheel and her hunched-over body how white her knuckles I might be. I followed her for about three miles between thinking to pass her and just staying behind her. All of a sudden she fishtailed a bit and went front-first into the ditch. Since her speed was so slow, she did not enter the ditch too far.

I stopped to see if I could be of assistance. An elderly women emerged from the car. I said, "What are you doing out on a day like this? I have to be out, but what is your reason?" She commented that her dog needed some food, and she needed garbage bags. I shook my head but made no further comment. She got back in the car, and with some effort on my part regarding pushing the front of the vehicle and her using the accelerator, we freed the car from the ditch.

I followed her to the grocery store in the next town with no further incidence. I applauded her bravery for taking on the road conditions, but I could not understand in my mind, her reasoning to be out in the elements just to get some food for her dog and some garbage bags.

When I returned down the same route, I did not see any indications she did not make it back home. I did wonder if she had family who checked in on her occasionally, or was the dog the only importance to her. I have found, as I am sure others have found, that first impressions when you first meet someone are not always positive. Sometimes a negative initial contact can continue to be negative after each meeting. Then again, the attitudes could change between both individuals.

Such was the case when I met a sewage disposal system installer for the first time in 1973. Jokester was on leave for training for the National Guard. I, therefore, was recruited to cover his area. A 3:00 p.m. Friday afternoon final inspection brought me to my first interaction with this installer. The man was in his mid-forties and he had two young sons who worked with him. I discovered afterword that he had been installing systems for several years. Many of the new regulations, I further discovered, were not to his liking. However, during his inspection, I was not aware of this information.

I introduced myself. He reciprocated my review of who I was and my background with the statement, "You're new aren't you?" I said, "Yes, that is why I introduced myself to you." I could see by his actions he was not impressed. I added to his disdain for me when I informed him I could not let him complete the installation by covering it, because he needed to make a few corrections to the system. He did not argue or appear to be upset with my conclusions; he just stared at me. I informed him that when the corrections were complete, someone would return to approve the corrections.

The following Monday, Jokester was back at work. I informed him of the details of my inspection. That afternoon, he followed up my inspection. I did not hear any feedback from Jokester regarding his attitude during that inspection.

About a week and a half later, my boss received a letter from the installer which stated that our department was going to "hell in a handbasket" because we were sending "snot-nosed kids" out to do services who only knew about inspecting restaurants. He further stated that the new regulations were bad enough but to send some horse's hind end out who was green as grass was too much to swallow. He added that he was done working in our county.

I told my boss that I did not feel I was a "snot-nosed kid," after all I was now twenty-five years old, and I also always tried to keep my nose clean. My boss said pay him no mind. He informed me that he crossed paths with him many times when the department inspected milk producer's operations during the 1950s. During these times, he could be rather caustic at times.

About two years later, I met again with him. He appeared to be accustomed to the requirements. I was summoned to develop a replacement sewage system for an existing piece of property. Upon my arrival, I discovered that the design of a system was going to require some complicated strategy. The location of the home, other structures, neighbor's wells, the owner's well, location of a lake, and the elevation of the property made for the need for some complicated design specifications. To my surprise, the installer did not comment regarding our first meeting, and I did not remind him, having sense to leave well enough alone. In fact, our coming together was very much the opposite. He complimented me on my clever and crafty method of solving the conundrum with which we were faced. After this meeting, we became rather comfortable with each other for several years. His thoughts and jargon and those of others will be the subject of the final chapter of this book.

# THE TALE END

AS I STATED IN THE introduction, I have always enjoyed the world of jokes and puns. I have also always been intrigued and curious about the use of idioms and catch phrases that are long-time popular and, on the other hand, short-term popular.

Sitting pretty, don't sell him or her short, shoot the breeze, pay through the nose, bend over backwards, shake a leg, get going, kick up my heels, knock yourself out, dirt cheap, take for granted, neck of the woods, far out, catty-corner, as the crow flies, a little hanky panky going on, coming to terms, don't make a lot of fuss and foofaraw, sharp as a serpent's tooth, cool as the center seed of a cucumber, yessiree Bob, got along swimmingly, has courage of his or her convictions, plain as the nose on your face, ball park figure, music has charm to soothe savage beast, live and let live, tickled pink, hands down, sick as a dog, till the cows come home, close but no cigar, rise and shine, raining cats and dogs, slap on the wrist, when pigs fly, hold your horses, loose cannon, keep your chin up, and much obliged, are some of the catch phrases that I have heard over the years on this planet we live on.

I heard these expressions many times from people I came in contact with on a daily basis at my job. I mention at the end of the last "tale" the sewage system installer who became a longtime acquaintance.

He was a man at times "set in his ways," but if you explained to him why something had to be accomplished a certain way with good reasoning, he would be a champion for the cause of public health protection and was a "godsend" for dealing with public. He was also helpful in dealing with difficult situations. As time went by, I realized he had a "gift for the gab." He had an accomplished jargon. When he felt someone was talking too much, he said, "It takes courage to stand in front of someone and speak, but it takes the same amount of fortitude to sit done and shut up and listen." Regarding the same subject, he said, "Old Indian proverb: talk little, listen much."

When he was faced with a tough situation, he said, "I will have to bite the tin foil and face the music." He said, "Change is permanent," when discussing new requirements.

Although I never saw or heard him get in an altercation, he said a number of times, "If you are a constant whiner, you may end up with a minor shiner."

He said, "Demographics are for dense people."

He said, "If you expect respect, be the first to show it."

He said, "My wife said I made some bad decisions; this was, of course, after I married her."

He said, "Work like you don't need the money, and you will not have the money when you need it."

He said to me, " Pick your battles wisely," and (battling with him was not wise).

He said, " Nothing worth working for was worth nothing without hard work." (That was "pretty much" my dad's belief.)

He said, " If you look back at what you have accomplished, you should experience satisfaction."

He always called his wife the "old heifer" when referring to her.

One sunny Saturday in 2006, I went to the evening Mass in another town. To my surprise, during the ceremony there was time set aside for the installer and his wife to repeat their marriage vows for their fiftieth anniversary. He even made some comments about his wife, after the ceremony. He said, "Anything worth doing should come with satisfaction after doing it. Marrying his wife was worth doing."

He said, "Only a life lived for others is a life worthwhile." He quoted Einstein a lot over the years. I asked him if the "worthwhile quote" was one of Albert's; he said indeed it was.

Another surprise was that after all the years of knowing him, the subject of being Catholic never came up.

Another character who stands out among many others who provided their own jargon was a chap who liked to share jokes. "Much obliged" was always his closing remark after you did something for him. I enjoyed those words because my dad and others always would say those words when I was young. You do not hear them much; they have "gone by the wayside.".

One of his favorite puns was, "The owner of a toupee company was a Big Wig." He asked me, "How do you make holy water? You boil the hell out of it"; and "Why were the Indians here first? They had reservations."

On a serious note he said," You learn as a toddler to talk, but silence comes with wisdom when you mature."

He said many times, "He thought if money came in the door and was not thought of correctly, happiness went out the door."

He said, "If you wish to poison youth, poison their entertainment."

He said, "If you want a friend, get a dog."

He said, "If you need a place to spend some time alone, go where no one else goes."

He said, "If you do something for others, it is remembered; if you cheat someone, it is also remembered."

Another idiom he said, after finishing a statement about a situation he was involved in was, "Well, the upshot of what happened was:" You do not hear the word "upshot" much anymore.

Many people influence us throughout life in the manner we conduct ourselves and the methods we follow to try to become successful. I remember reading a thought not too long ago; I do not know who I can attribute it to and I do not know if it is exactly as I read it, but it went something like this:

The road to life can be rough, but do not give up. You may have setbacks. You may need to start over. You may need to change your method of living, but don't give up. Just find another direction to take with what you have left to work with after the setback.

My folks spoke a lot about Mahatma Ghandi when I was young. One of my favorite quotes of his is the following:

Keep your thoughts positive, because your thoughts become your words.

Keep your words positive, because your words become your behavior.

Keep your behavior positive, because your behavior becomes your habits.

Keep your habits positive, because your habits become your values.

Keep your values positive, because your values become your destiny.

This is the "Tale End."

CPSIA information can be obtained
at www.ICGtesting.com
Printed in the USA
FFHW011530030219
50356007-55455FF